A Nutrition Revolution

A Nutrition Revolution

Elizabeth Kahn

First published by AuthorHouse 09/19/2011

ISBN: 978-1-4634-2470-1 (sc)
ISBN: 978-1-4634-2471-8 (hc)
ISBN: 978-1-4634-2469-5 (ebk)

Library of Congress Control Number: 2011911047

Reprinted with IngramSpark   02/13/2019

ISBN: 978-1-73363-17-0-9 (sc)

Contents

i.   Foreword

I remember my pediatrician. I remember the sterile white floors, the crunchy tissue-like paper that covered the patient table, and the freezing cold temperatures of the examination room. When I was sick as a child, I distinctly remember being horrified at the thought of having to leave my house, go to the doctor, put on the patient gown and freeze while he listened to my lungs, swabbed my throat and tapped around my joints to check my reflexes. But more than the décor, the climate and the crackling paper, I most often recall my pediatrician for his characteristic treat at the end of the visit: the lollipops.

To ease the pain and panic of any kid's trip to the doctor, my pediatrician always had a jar full of lollipops. Little white sticks topped with (undoubtedly) artificial colors, flavors, sweeteners, and corn syrup, colorfully displayed in a clear canister to entice all of us resistant children. But why wouldn't we love to visit a practitioner who made us feel better? Maybe it was because what was making us sick could have been healed with fewer trips to the doctor and more outings to the farmer's market; a little less penicillin and a few more plants. Throughout my research at John F. Kennedy University's Master's program in holistic health education and nutrition, I became acutely aware of this country's psychological dependence on pharmaceuticals as the "only" means of healing and health. Even children are taught at a young age that if something is "wrong," only a doctor and drugs can fix it. Elizabeth Kahn's *A Nutrition Revolution* exposes the misinformation that consumers receive from food manufacturers, drug corporations and the diet industry: information that tells us that junk food and diets are what we need and that drugs cure illness.

But the whistle has been blown on food, drug and diet companies in the past, which is why Elizabeth Kahn's work delves deeper. The overwhelming evidence about the corruption in our food system is only the beginning. Without workable resolutions, we are left with a dismal outlook on our health and current health-care system. Elizabeth Kahn's *A Nutrition Revolution* gives us the real "active ingredients" for nursing ourselves back to health: nutrition. When we ingest nutrients instead of popping pills—and seek nutrition guidance instead of our "doctor's orders"—we can heal ourselves and experience sustainable health.

Our health in America is on life support. We spend trillions of dollars every year on healthcare ($2 trillion in 2006), yet obesity, heart disease, autoimmune disorders, diabetes and Attention Deficit Disorder (ADD) continue to climb up the chart of concerns. We need to pull the plug on the current focus of health—from pharmaceuticals to nutrition, which is what *A Nutrition Revolution* does.

Elizabeth Kahn is at the forefront of a paradigm shift: a re-shifting of focus toward root causes like nutrition and education. If you are a parent, an educator, or even a policy maker, this book is a must-read for you to empower yourselves, your children, your students, and your community. Elizabeth Kahn challenges us to take health into our own hands; to realize that nutrition is the most cost-effective, most health-sustaining and most powerful anti-inflammatory, cholesterol-lowering, anti-cancer, anti-aging "product" in the market today (grocery market, that is).

When I have given nutrition talks to clients, parents and educators, I was always looking for one resource to recommend that succinctly explained food politics while providing tangible, user-friendly ideas for change. Elizabeth Kahn's *A Nutrition Revolution* is that guide that will now be at the top of my recommended reading list.

The time of dragging our children to the doctor whenever something is less than perfect is a thing of the past. We have the tools to be proactive health experts; to heal ourselves with the items in our refrigerator. Let's start enticing our children less with colorful lollipops at the doctor's office. It is time to introduce them to a new rainbow of colors . . . the ones you find neatly stacked around the produce section of your local grocery store.

Jaime L. Mitchell
Masters of Arts, Holistic Health Education, specialization in Holistic Nutrition
Publisher & Owner of *Natural Awakenings Magazine,* East Bay
Founder of Healthy **SOUL**utions

ii.   Introduction

"No army can withstand the strength of an idea whose time has come."—*Victor Hugo*

Since my body was healed and life changed with nutrition, my mission has been to spread the word and help others heal naturally.

This book contains answers to questions I am asked most often, like, "Why did you become a nutritionist?" "How were *you* healed?" "Why doesn't my doctor know more about nutrition?" "Why won't my insurance plan pay for nutrition consulting?" "How can I get my child to eat more vegetables?" "Are carbohydrates bad for you?" "What do you think about this food or that diet fad?"

These pages contain the information needed to implement changes in our doctors' offices, voting booths, grocery stores, homes and schools, and to make the necessary shifts in our attitudes and priorities about nutrition.

This is not another "how to diet" book. This is a "how to understand nutrition" book. It is about *education* and making a philosophical shift in our approach to health.

The reader will not only learn about nutrition, but also a formula to repair our struggling health and healthcare, political, economic and education systems. We must dig deep to resolve our health and other issues and *that* is what *A Nutrition Revolution* does.

This work has been designed for all people, but especially for consumers, voters and those in public policy-making positions. For those of you who know, deep down, there *has* to be a better way, this is for you.

Road Map to Reading *A Nutrition Revolution*

The reader will be taken down the same path that led to my good health and will become empowered, as I was, to heal themselves and others.

The original title was *Kids, Nutrition and Learning* but eventually evolved into *A Nutrition Revolution* in order to encompass the entire problem, which is systemic and deeply embedded into the U.S. psyche and culture.

The subject matter is now applicable to those of all ages. There is still a lot of information on child nutrition, education and how nutrients affect the brain, but also on Western medicine, diet and the American culture, advertising, supply and demand, lobbying, politics, nutrition fundamentals and food manufacturing.

A Nutrition Revolution is divided into three main parts: the problems, proof, and solutions. Hypotheses were developed, data collected, conclusions drawn and findings presented. The roots of the problems have been located, uprooted, examined and exposed to the light — as *that* is the most effective way to solve any problem.

This information is not entirely new, but has been put together to lead the way out of the quagmire this country and many of its residents are currently in.

The words on these pages are not "sugar-coated" because our society has been glazing over these issues and looking for quick fixes for far too long. Now, it is time for some *real* answers. The reader will gain many of those answers, a nutrition *education* and will know how to proceed to the next step of what we must do.

We must begin *A Nutrition Revolution.*

Acknowledgements

I have had much spiritual guidance along my healing and learning path—and in writing this book—and want to thank God for His support.

Thank you to my parents who have supported me and told me I could do anything—I believed you. Thank you to my friends and family for being infinitely understanding and patient during the past several years.

Thank you, Sonia, for healing me; Kelly for helping me get these words down on paper. Without either of you this book may not have been written. Thanks to all of the other contributors to this book including Amy, Doreen, Jaime and Ross; bless you all.

Chapter One

My Story

"Eat an apple on going to bed, and you'll keep the doctor from earning his bread." – English proverb

A Mystery

Years ago, I felt sick, and like most people do when they're sick, went to doctors for help. After several tests, they told me there was nothing wrong with me. I was sure they were wrong. My undiagnosed symptoms included headaches, insomnia, moodiness and fatigue. The doctors did find one problem, however. One doctor told me my frequent stomachaches may be due to lactose intolerance and suggested I take a pill.

Some time earlier, my neighbor, a nutritionist, told me everyone should see a nutritionist at least once in their lives. I remembered that advice and 'eenie meenie miney moe'd' in the phonebook to find one. I went to see her, even though my insurance only paid $20 of the $80-per-visit charge.

An Awakening

During my first visit, the nutritionist asked about my symptoms and asked me to keep a food journal. During the next few visits, she continually modified my diet until the right one was found and my symptoms disappeared.

The nutritionist agreed that I was lactose intolerant, but also said I had other food allergies and an intestinal yeast buildup. She told me I was consuming too much white flour, suggested several dietary changes and a cleansing regimen. All of this helped put my body back into balance, naturally.

The difference between the doctors' and the nutritionist's philosophies can best be described by their approaches to my lactose intolerance. The doctor suggested I take a lactose pill whenever I ate dairy. The nutritionist suggested I remove the source of the problem, cow's milk.

Many of the changes my nutritionist suggested were simple — substitutions like using almond milk or soymilk and eating cultured dairy products that are easier to digest, like yogurt and cottage cheese; eating more fruits and vegetables; consuming fewer processed foods; and how to eat in a more balanced way. It was more than worth the $60 out-of-pocket expense because, within months, my symptoms were gone.

Even though drugs and doctors' visits were covered under my insurance plan, they could not help me stabilize my body *before* it broke. The nutritionist did, with only paper, pencil and healthy food.

The money that both my insurance company and I saved on more doctors' visits, tests, medication and "special" diet food is undeniable. My private nutrition crash course cost me about $700, but also saved me future medical expenses and the inconvenience of developing major health issues like hypothyroidism, diabetes or hypoglycemia, of which I was having symptoms.

If I had not been healed through better nutrition, I probably would have ended up on medications and suffered from their unpleasant side effects. The alterations in my diet did cause so-called side effects: increased energy, better moods; healthier hair and skin; and other health improvements I didn't even know were related. I not only felt 100 percent better, but even lost ten pounds to reach my ideal weight.

While searching for answers, I became frustrated with the doctors. One of them noticed this and explained that they often have to wait for things to break to treat them. She said the body is strong and can hold out for a while, but will eventually break down under continued pressure, and *then* problems will show up on a test.

While I was dealing with my health issues, I bounced back and forth between doctors and nutritionists and passed messages between them. In the end, this process worked, but I had to research it, hand-hold it and pay for it. It would have been more efficient if care-givers would have shared information directly and nutrition was acknowledged more by Western medicine.

A History

Diabetes runs in my family. Dietary habits, like genes, can be passed down. Both play a role in our bodies, but, in our society, the former is often overlooked.

During my childhood, I ate home-cooked meals with vegetables every day with one parent — and doughnuts, Taco Bell and candy every other weekend with the other. My dad would send me to the doughnut store with $20 and my three sisters on Saturday morning. Probably to stop us from jumping on the bed and waking him up. My sisters and I went wide-eyed to Winchell's doughnut house and bought the store. My mother, on the other hand, made us sit down to dinner every night and eat our vegetables.

I learned about the value of food from both of my parents — the fun from my dad and the function from my mom. But guess which side of my family has diabetes? You guessed it: the doughnut eaters. Eating doughnuts and Taco Bell once in a while is not a problem, but eating these unhealthy foods all the time *does* cause problems — including diabetes.

My health problems did not start until after I moved out and was on my own. My favorite foods were Cap'n Crunch cereal and macaroni and cheese. This eventually took a toll and, in my late twenties, I started to feel and look sick. Luckily, I found out it was my diet and quickly altered it to feel better.

Since learning how to balance my body chemistry through nutrition, I mainly crave healthy food, and not junk food, anymore. Now I can still eat an occasional doughnut — and who doesn't want to do that? But I also like to make and eat healthy foods like smoothies and salads and feel the burst of energy afterward.

Another profound moment happened while watching a television news program about Attention Deficit Disorder (ADD) and diet. The show's reporters followed two children diagnosed with ADD. One boy was treated at a drug camp where doctors experimented with different drugs. At one point, the boy, apparently reacting to the drugs, was standing still, staring into space, and repeatedly sticking his tongue in and out. In another instance, he was screaming and throwing a tantrum.

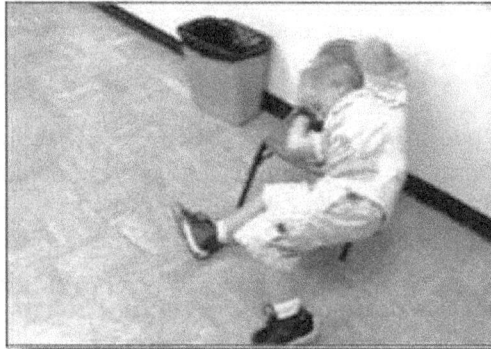

Out of Control

The news program followed another boy to a nutrition specialist. He tested positive for dietary imbalances and food allergies and, after receiving diet therapy, was able to get off of his medications.[1] Many of my symptoms were the same as the ones those children suffered from.

This program was the catalyst for what would be a major life transformation for me. I was already convinced about nutrition's role in disorders like ADD, but was so moved by this particular program that I called a college counselor the next day to pursue a nutrition degree.

A Mission

Four and a half years of intensive study and a $180,000 education later, I have become empowered and can now take charge of my own health and life, and can help others do the same. While not everyone needs a four-year science degree in nutrition, everyone should have a basic nutrition education.

My first degree was in *clinical* nutrition—which involves a lot of chemistry. I learned there are millions of simultaneous chemical reactions occurring in our bodies all the time fueled and catalyzed by nutrition, the connection between food and our bodies.

Nutrition is not wizardry, but trying to find a job in prevention and natural healing was. After graduating, I had three basic choices: become a registered dietitian (RD) and work for a hospital formulating tube feedings, work for a school district planning lunch menus (choosing between french fries and tater tots), or counsel poor pregnant women about nutrition. But if a nutrition graduate like me wants work in natural healing or educating mainstream society about nutrition, good luck!

If I would have completed the registered dietitian program, I could have made a career in one of the positions I just mentioned and made a decent salary, but that was not what I wanted to do. I wanted to keep people healthy and out of the hospital and treat those who were already sick naturally.

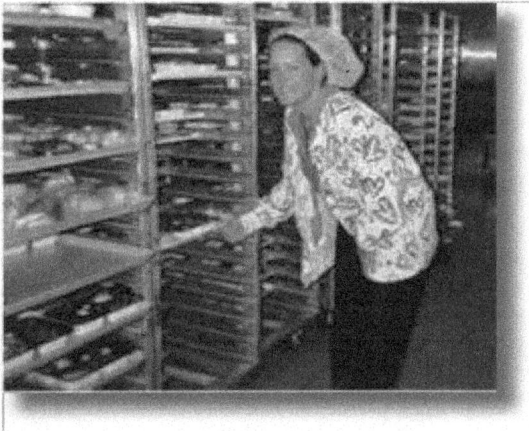

Hospital Menu Planning

After much persistence, re-enrolling in school for a second degree in education, volunteering in positions I sought, and searching for work for several years, I finally found a job in nutrition education *and* natural healing. I now teach nutrition in an elementary school and have a nutrition consulting practice.

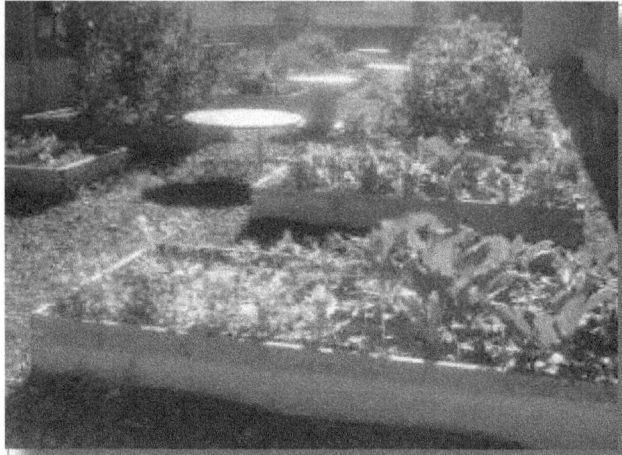

My Classroom

I did not take the path most traveled—or the one of least resistance. I instead fought and blazed a trail and am now a nutrition counselor, teacher and writer. I can spread the word about nutrition, treat people naturally and help keep people healthy as I wanted to do.

Even though nutrition can prevent and treat disease, the availability of nutrition information in this country is severely lacking. This is not due to a lack of demand, as many people want this information. Many are frustrated and are seeking answers. What we lack is the infrastructure to provide these answers. Jobs in nutrition education and natural healing must be made more available. This book is designed to light the way and open more doors in the field of nutrition so we can all heal.

Chapter Two

Medicine

"It is only the inferior physician who treats the illness he was unable to prevent." – Chinese medical proverb

You feel sick, so you go to the doctor — if you're lucky enough to afford one these days. The response you will likely get from that doctor is:

"I don't know what causes your problem or how to fix it, but here is a pill for your symptoms. It will probably cause side effects. If this doesn't work, we can eventually remove the malfunctioning organ and try more pills." Or one of these:

"You have diabetes; I can put you on diabetes medication."

"Your thyroid has given out; I can put you on thyroid medication."

"You are morbidly obese; I can recommend you for gastric bypass surgery."

"Your cholesterol is high; I can put you on cholesterol medication."

The problem with these approaches is that they place an undue importance on treating *symptoms* rather than root causes. A symptom is just the body's way of saying something is wrong. Doctors don't listen to symptoms to find their origin; instead, they try to subdue them with powerful drugs that cause even more problems. Surgery is not ideal either, as surgery removes body parts *after* they have broken. Nutrition eliminates symptoms by addressing root causes — which are often diet related — and keeps body parts from breaking and other problems from arising due to drugs' further impact on an already imbalanced body chemistry.

Pills vs. Plants

In medicine, when a substance is discovered that treats a condition or symptom, it is isolated, concentrated and prescribed to the patient. Problem solved, right? Wrong. This simplistic approach not only ignores the ultimate root cause but also the complicated, delicate balance of chemicals within our bodies.

Drugs cause side effects, which are often listed at the end of drug commercials. The commentator's voice calmly says something like:

"Side effects may include rash, skin discoloration, itching, swelling, wheezing, coughing, choking, thoughts of suicide . . ."

Here are some *actual* side effects caused by a common blood-thinning medication:

> *Side effects can include: Nausea, vomiting, loss of appetite, stomach or abdominal bloating or cramps, serious bleeding, pain, swelling, discomfort, prolonged bleeding from cuts or gums, persistent nosebleeds, unusually heavy or prolonged menstrual flow, bruising, dark urine, black stools, severe headache, dizziness, nausea, vomiting, abdominal pain, yellowing of eyes or skin. This drug can cause serious (possibly fatal) complications from the dislodging of solid patches of cholesterol from blood vessel walls, which can block the blood supply to parts of the body and can cause severe tissue damage and gangrene. Other symptoms include painful red rash, dark discoloration of any body part, purple toe syndrome, sudden intense pain, back or muscle pain, foot ulcers, change in the amount of urine, vision changes, confusion, slurred speech, one-sided weakness, rash, itching, swelling, severe dizziness, trouble breathing and more.*[1]

Many nutrients can thin the blood. According to popular alternative medical practitioner Dr. Andrew Weil, M.D., there are many natural substances that are blood thinners, but no studies have compared their effectiveness to pharmaceutical blood thinners.

Historically, many foods have been used as medicine. In fact, many of today's drugs come from nature. Penicillin, the first antibiotic, comes from the mold of corn and cantaloupe. Herbs are plants that are used as medicine and can treat many health problems. Kava root, for example, can treat anxiety. St. John's wort can alleviate depression.

Aspirin came from a plant, but is only part of the plant that is, like other drugs, manipulated and concentrated. Aspirin can relieve pain and thin the blood but also causes stomach problems and excessive bleeding. Meadowsweet, the first plant in which salicylic acid was discovered, and from which aspirin was later synthesized, is an organic pain reliever and fever reducer that does not cause the harmful side-effects aspirin does.[2] We should listen to Mother Nature more instead of continually trying to improve upon her work — as she has always had the answers.

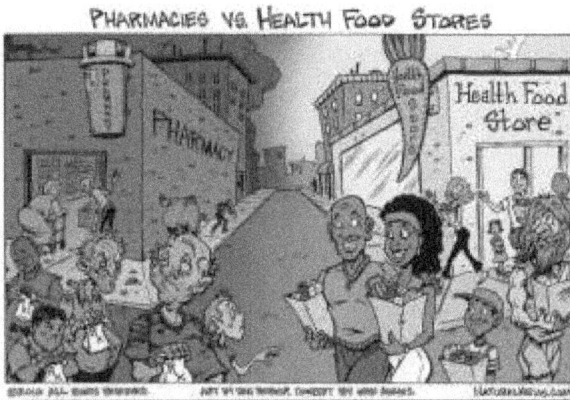

Drug Money

The pharmaceutical industry, also known as "big pharma," is — year after year — one of the most profitable industries.[3] The legal drug trade brings in 300 billion dollars a year in the U.S. alone and 650 billion dollars globally.[4, 5]

A billion dollars seems like a mythical number, so let's break it down: one billion dollars is equal to one-thousand million dollars. Does that help? Basically, *a lot* of U.S. dollars are being spent on drugs.

Pharmaceutical companies are most likely not trying to find cures for disease or trying to prevent them because doing so will not benefit them financially. If people stay sick and get sicker, they will need more pills and the companies and shareholders will make money, which is their ultimate goal.

Here is what the ten top-selling drugs make annually:

1. Lipitor for cholesterol: $14 billion

2. Advair for asthma: $6 billion

3. Plavix for cardiovascular disease: $6 billion

4. Nexium for stomach acidity, ulcers and reflux disease (GERD): $5 billion

5. Norvasc for high blood pressure and angina pain: $5 billion

6. Remicade for autoimmune disorders like rheumatoid arthritis: $4 billion

7. Enbrel for autoimmune diseases like rheumatoid arthritis: $4 billion

8. Zyprexa for schizophrenia and bipolar disorder: $4 billion

9. Diovan for high blood pressure and congestive heart failure: $4 billion

10. Risperdal for schizophrenia: $4 billion[6]

COUNTERTHINK

"RACE FOR THE CURE"

CANCER INDUSTRY

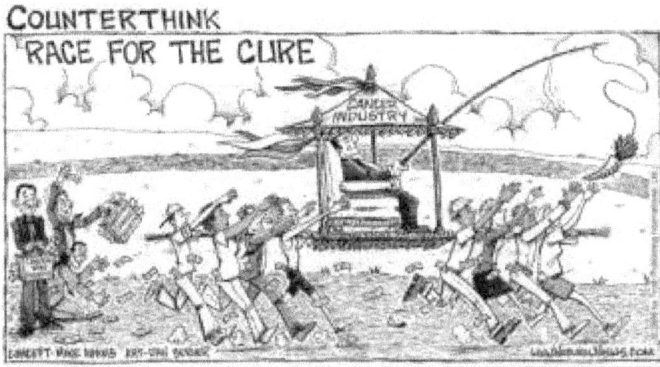

Cholesterol medications are the drug industry's biggest money-makers. Spinach, one of the most nutrient-dense foods out there, can heal the body in many ways—including lowering cholesterol. Spinach has an annual farm value of 175 million dollars—which is about one percent of the money made from just one brand of cholesterol medication.[6, 7]

Blood-thinning medications are the second-largest selling class of drug on the market today. New blood-thinners are expected to bring in ten billion dollars a year by 2015.[8] Vitamin E—found in foods like almonds and algae—can also thin the blood. Almonds make up a large chunk of U.S. agriculture revenue. Almond production was recently at a rare, almost all-time high of $1.7 billion a year.[9] But this is still only a fraction, about one-sixth, of blood-thinning drug revenue.

Erectile dysfunction (ED) can be cured with diet—and with amino acids in particular.[10, 11] One brand of ED medication, Viagra, earned a half of a billion dollars in one quarter in 2009.[12] A bottle of ED pills costs from $100 to $200. On the other hand, whole-foods, rich in amino acids, cost a lot less.

Diet intervention can be used to treat, and even cure, many mental disorders. But in one report, researchers state that nutritional therapies have become a "long-forgotten method of treatment" in mental disorders because the drug companies have no interest in something they cannot patent or own.[13] There is more on this in The Brain chapter.

If people ate more healthy foods including almonds, spinach and algae, there would also be fewer incidences of diabetes and obesity, two of our society's largest health epidemics. But there isn't nearly as much money in farming spinach, almonds or algae as there is in blood-thinning, diabetes, cholesterol, obesity, ED or psychopharmacologic medications. This financial disparity is perpetuating the drug vs. nutrition problem and is why there is more access to drugs than nutrition information in this country.

Healthcare

We have a reason to fix our problems. Our healthcare system is in financial ruins. The U.S. spent over two trillion dollars on healthcare in 2007 — thirty times the amount it did in 1970 — but Americans' health is only getting worse.[14, 15]

Healthcare costs rose from $4,000 per person to $8,000 between 1998 and 2008, and these costs continue to rise.[14] By the year 2015, healthcare costs are expected to increase to $13,000 per person, more than triple the amount they were in 1998. The U.S. is ranked thirty-seventh in health outcome worldwide. It spends nearly twice as much per capita as any industrialized country, but has a lower life expectancy. For the first time, children are now projected to have a shorter lifespan than their parents. The U.S. medical system is broken because it sets out to manage, not prevent, end-stage disease.[16]

Cost Savings

Nutrition has been proven to save money on healthcare costs, but, right now, nutritionists are a luxury most cannot afford. Doctors and drugs are extensively covered by all major health plans, and, although at least as effective, nutritionists and healthy food are not.

One study found that, if Medicare beneficiaries with high blood pressure received nutrition therapy, healthcare costs over a five-year period could be cut by an estimated 52 million dollars.[17] If diet therapy were applied to even more diseases, the savings could be billions or even trillions of dollars.

Medical School

Doctors do not understand nutrition because they are not trained in it. Many only receive a two-hour nutrition lecture in medical school. Doctors *are* taught about pharmaceutical and surgical solutions, however. Perhaps it is no coincidence, then, that roughly 20 percent of medical schools' yearly budgets comes from the drug industry.[18]

More than half of graduating medical students say their nutrition preparation was inadequate.[19] Some doctors say what little bit of nutrition education they do receive is quite often wrong. Medical students say professors aren't talking about nutrition — and pharmaceutical companies aren't, either. The impression these doctors get during medical school is that if it isn't being taught, it must not be important. But they *are* taught vitamin deficiencies can cause diseases like beriberi and pellagra; however, a doctor who prescribes vitamins to his or her patients is viewed by their counterparts as a "quack".[20]

In this country we don't teach nutrition to doctors and do not offer it to most of the sick, yet we provide a nutritionist to every patient in the hospital. When a patient is very ill or near death, we finally acknowledge nutrition works? This is too little too late. Everyone should have access to a nutritionist at the first sign of a health problem to keep their bodies from breaking and ending up in the hospital at all.

Convenient Controversy

The top two most profitable industries are the oil and pharmaceutical industries.[3] Do you think it is a coincidence then that both global warming and natural healing are controversial? The common denominators in both of these industries are that they are extremely profitable and opposition to them is controversial.

Deliberate controversy designed purely for financial gain may seem implausible *but* former corporate executives have reported they *did* participate in corporate smear campaigns against those who would negatively impact their profits.[21]

There are Websites entirely dedicated to discrediting natural cures and practitioners. One Website, "Quackwatch.com," does not call Western medicine or pharmaceuticals "quackery"; instead, they consistently call natural supplements and practitioners quacks. They do seem to have only one-dimensional opinions.

If Quackwatch were being fair, it might mention how medications often do not work and even cause death. Quackwatch has its own credibility issues. The founder has had lawsuits filed against him, had his lawsuits thrown out of court, and, according to a rebuttal from one of his human "targets," does not hold a valid medical license or a nutrition science degree.[22, 23]

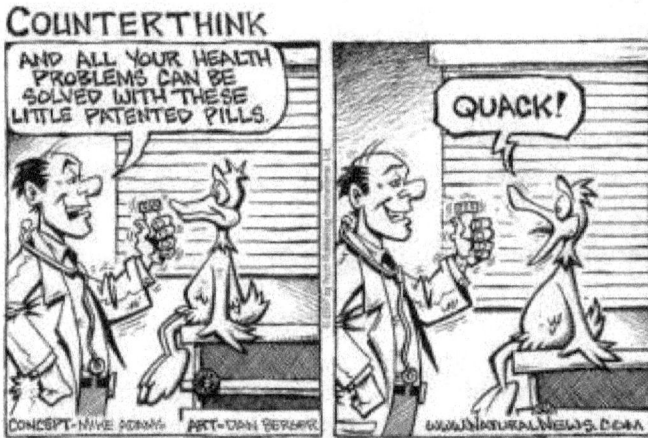

Drug Promotion

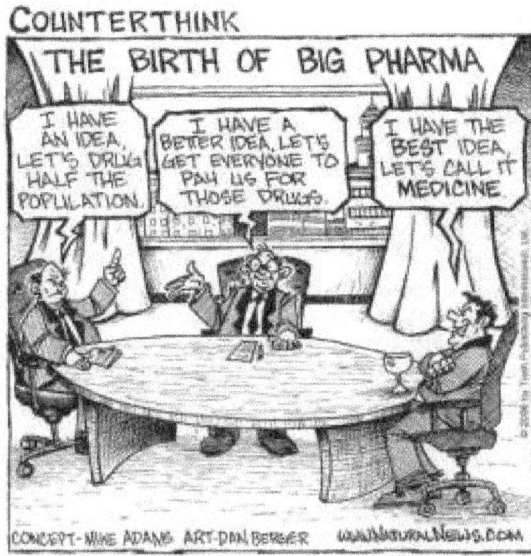

The drug companies are strategic in selling their products. The pharmaceutical industry spends more money on lobbying than any other industry. They spent 855 million dollars between 1998 and 2006 on lobbying.[24] That money was meant to encourage legislation in Congress to benefit their financial bottom line.

In addition to promoting themselves to lawmakers, drug companies also promote themselves to doctors and the public. In 2005, the pharmaceutical industry spent over four billion dollars on direct-to-consumer advertising and seven billion dollars on professional promotion.[25] And it works. Doctors give drugs to patients for all of their ailments, and patients often inquire about—or demand to receive—medications they've seen advertised on T.V.

Some are even being accused of "disease-mongering" in order to maximize profits. In one paper, researchers state that "coming years will bear greater witness to the corporate-sponsored creation of disease."[26] Sickness should not be for-profit; perhaps, instead wellness should be.

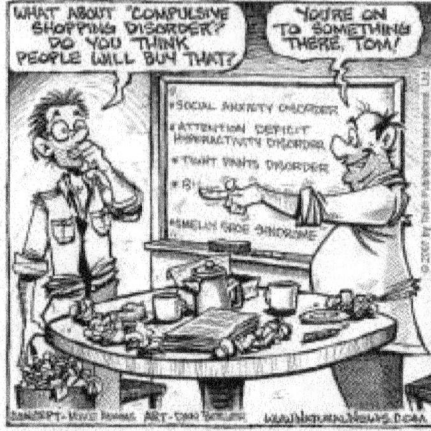

Alternative Medicine

When Western doctors and natural practitioners work together, it is called alternative, complementary or integrated medicine. Natural practitioners include naturopathic doctors, nutritionists, chiropractors, acupuncturists and more.

If I were in a car accident and in need of emergency surgery, I'd want to be under the care of a good surgeon. On the other hand, if I was diagnosed with cancer, I would head straight to an alternative care facility — presuming I could find and afford one.

The idea behind conventional medicine is to create a hostile environment for the disease in the body, so it cannot thrive — called "allopathy". Many drugs and surgeries create a hostile environment in the body, all right. Take cancer, for instance, one of the most common diseases today. The key characteristic of cancer is that some cells in the body keep dividing; they do not know when to stop. This uncontrolled cell division is what creates tumors. Cell division is one of the most important and fundamental life processes. But in cancer, this process has gone awry. Chemotherapy, the most common cancer treatment, is designed to kill these out-of-control cells with powerful chemicals. Patients who undergo chemotherapy feel near death because that is literally what is happening. Doctors, of course, have to stop prior to the patient actually dying, but death is the idea behind chemotherapy treatment.

There are many proven and promising natural treatments for cancer and other diseases, like diet therapy, that are not harsh or invasive, but they are not being researched or taken seriously enough by Western medicine.[27]

Natural medicine works to stimulate the body's own immune system and natural defenses by supporting the body so it can heal itself, which it is designed to do. Natural healing is the opposite approach of "allopathy".

These comprehensive health programs must be incorporated into mainstream medicine for our society to progress and achieve optimal health.

What Western medicine, the healthcare system, and our bodies need are more effective and low-cost solutions, like nutrition. But for this to happen, patients must educate themselves. If patients learn more about natural methods, they will be able to say, "No, thank you, Doctor," as I was able to do.

Chapter Three

Society

"Let us eat and drink, for tomorrow we diet." — Wendy Morgan

Our society is preyed upon by the food, drug and diet industries. We are becoming fatter, sicker and more medicated. Our quality of life is deteriorating. We are in a cycle of poor health, decreasing education levels and a boom-to-bust economy. This is a snowball of failure that is only getting bigger — continually gaining momentum — and we must intervene to stop it. We need the right tools to fix these problems, and one of those tools is nutrition.

How do you feel after a healthy meal? Energetic, clear-minded, focused? Ready to take on the world? How would you feel after a day of chips and soda? This is the difference between healthy and unhealthy food.

Unhealthy food is practically all that is available, and affordable, in certain (by that, read "poor") areas. There are a disproportionate number of poor people who are sick due to diet-related illnesses. An unhealthy diet has a negative impact on learning and education — and education levels often determine financial stability and success.[1, 2]

Most people in this country eat poorly, feel sick and believe drugs or diets can fix their problems. But the masses are only responding to what they are told over and over. On television, there are back-to-back commercials for fast and junk food, diet food and drugs for everything a poor diet causes.

Have you ever tried yourself — or tried to get a child — to eat healthy regularly? If you are like most people, you probably found this to be a challenge. There are many reasons for that. Advertising is a big one, as I just mentioned. Children see an average of 10,000 junk food commercials a year. If parents spent every meal with their child, that would amount to only one-tenth of what television commercials expose them to. To make matters worse, fast-food companies have celebrities like Paris Hilton working for them. Parents and their healthy offerings have to compete with Hilton's, Britney Spears', Michael Jordan's and other attractive celebrities' not-so-healthy offerings.[3] Adding to the problem is that many people today are busy, struggling financially and there are cheap, fast and easy drive-through restaurants on practically every corner, with plenty of fatty, salty, sugary comfort food inside.

Junk food can cause fatigue. Many people today consume junk food then large energy drinks loaded with sugar, caffeine and other stimulating substances for a quick pick-me-up, but these products only add to the problem and further the chemical imbalances already going on inside the body.

Basically, all of the Happy Meals, fries, sodas, flaming hot chips, energy drinks and caramel macchiatos have caught up with us. Diets and drugs are not working, and our bodies are crumbling under the pressure. We don't need another wonder diet, "new and improved" energy drink or fancy medication—what we need is to fix the original problem—poor diet.

Flunking is expensive. Every year in the U.S., a lot of money is funneled into ventures of failure like junk and diet foods, prescription drugs, healthcare (or, more properly named, "sick care") and societal safety nets like welfare, prison, and war.

Spending on Failure
- Fast food: $200 billion[4]
- Diets: $50 billion[5]
- Drugs: $300 billion[6]
- Healthcare: $2 trillion[7]
- Prison: $200 billion[8]
- Welfare: $500 billion[9]
- War: $125 billion[10]

That is about three and a half *trillion* dollars spent on failing. We spend a fraction of this amount, one-sixth, on what we know leads to success: education.[11] One of the arguments used against education is that there is not enough money. This list proves that, yes, there *is* money; it just needs to be reinvested more wisely.

Reinvesting some of that money into more effective ventures like education, specifically nutrition education, will create another snowball effect—but a positive one, because nutrition education leads to better health, which leads to improvements in learning and education; higher education levels lead to more successful and productive people; more productive people paying into the system will lead to greater revenue and taxes as opposed to more sick, less educated people taking money out of the system via public healthcare, welfare, prison and other taxpayer-supported safety nets.

Many people across the globe fight wars for food and security. Seeds and classrooms are cheaper than bombs. We need to change our philosophy and approach to problems.

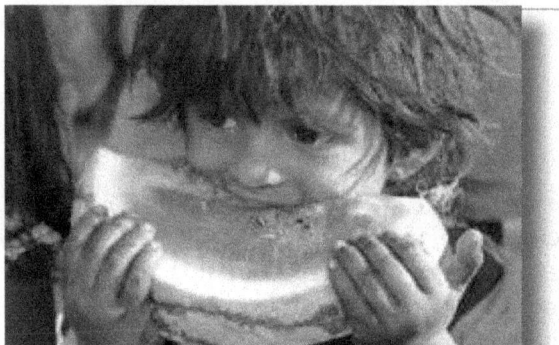

Hungry and Poor

The Opposition

As I have mentioned, there are people who try to discredit alternative methods for healing our society's poor health. I ran across some critics in an online discussion about plans for vegetable gardening in vacant inner-city lots—a type of program that has seen success in neighboring cities. These programs are inexpensive and they work. Studies show participants in garden nutrition programs eat more healthy foods.[12]

These critics said gardens were a costly waste of time and money. I responded to them and said that dirt and seeds are cheap. One of the commenters responded and said, "The soil is toxic." I explained that these types of gardens are built in raised beds using fresh, non-toxic soil. Plus, soil can be tested for toxicity. There are also plants (like sunflowers) that can absorb toxins.[13, 14] He basically called me an idiot and sent me a link about soil toxicity. I understand toxicity; I have studied it.

The fact is that many corporations will lose money, and maybe even go out of business, if the public gets healthy. As a result, these corporations may, in fact, be creating campaigns *against* nutrition. Is it possible that corporations may be participating in fighting the implementation of better nutrition because it will help their bottom lines? Of course it is.

Why is it such a social faux pas to use the term "conspiracy theory", when there are, today, many proven "conspiracies" in industry and government? A conspiracy is two or more people planning to do something illegal. Does what I have described sound like a far-fetched "conspiracy theory"?

Freedom of speech is an important right, but if someone is paid to spout an opinion simply to support an agenda, well that is called "propaganda" and I believe it happens in this country more often than most people realize. Regardless of whether or not these negative campaigners are being paid, *are* committing a crime or are just voicing their own opinions, they are in the way of progress by spreading uneducated opinions that many people believe.

The Solution

Our problems will not fix themselves. We will remain stuck in this cycle of perpetual failure if we continue with our current strategy — or lack thereof. Our strategy should be to focus on problems and address their root causes.

Nutrition is a viable and cost-effective solution to many of our health, societal and economic problems. Proponents of nutrition can win the arguments if they stand up and argue *persistently*.

So what can you do? Pay attention to current events. Fact-check what you see, hear and read. Research candidates, legislation and corporations. Vote with your voices, dollars and ballots. Heal yourself with nutrition—or other alternative means—and support preventative measures like nutrition education. Then shout it from the rooftops: "I want a nutrition revolution!"

Chapter Four

Politics

The U.S. has been hijacked by greed. Our own complacency has allowed those bent on achieving mass wealth at any cost to commandeer this nation. Our political and economic systems have lost their way. The original designs have eroded and all that is left are shells of what they once were.

It is often said, "The root of all evil is the love of money." This is because money equals *power* on this planet – and some want it obsessively.

We can fix what is broken, but first we must see the problem.

In capitalism, the key rule of supply and demand works – *if* it is allowed to flow freely and is unimpeded by dishonest manipulation. For example, consumers have wanted alternative-fueled vehicles for some time so the demand existed. But supply was denied to the market probably due to corporate interests and corresponding legislation. But if demand truly dictated the supply in the market, as it was designed to do, more alternative vehicles would have been built immediately in response to that demand.

As is the case with manipulated supply, a hindrance in natural demand also causes problems in the capitalistic model. Right now, food manufacturers are simply responding to a lack of demand for healthy food because the public is unaware of nutrition. If more people knew about nutrition, they would demand more healthy food. Suppliers would then create a supply and prices would go down. The missing part of the equation, though, is consumer awareness about nutrition. No doubt, largely, because some want to keep this information in the dark to continue to supply drugs – and then junk food to necessitate those drugs.

A competitive marketplace is also important in capitalism. If corporations become too large or monopolies occur, there is less competition and companies can then set their own prices or "price fix".

For capitalism to work, it must be properly regulated and monitored. Even some former executives of banks who were bailed out by the government in 2008 agree.[1]

The U.S. has an agency designed to watch over financial dealings — the Securities and Exchange Commission (SEC). But, many say the SEC is lacking adequate resources to sufficiently carry out its role; others allege corruption within the SEC.[2]

There are agencies designed to protect the consumer from unsafe foods and drugs. The Food and Drug Administration (FDA) is responsible for ensuring drugs, medical products, food products and other consumer goods are safe for the American public. The FDA regulates more than one trillion dollars in products, almost ten percent of the country's Gross Domestic Product. But, like the SEC, the FDA is said to be underfunded and overworked by wealthy private companies.

There are also allegations of corruption at the FDA. In 2009, FDA scientists stated that management is "corrupted and distorted" and that they "ordered, intimidated and coerced FDA experts to modify scientific evaluations, conclusions and recommendations in violation of the laws, rules and regulations, and to accept clinical and technical data that is not scientifically valid."[3]

In 1997, the FDA relaxed its guidelines for drug advertisements to the public. Since that time, spending on direct-to-consumer advertising by drug companies has risen dramatically — from $800 million to $4 billion a year in 2004, but staffing at the agency has not kept pace. The FDA has since been unable to keep up with and monitor all of the ads.[4]

The FDA has admitted their limited resources could result in delayed reviews of drug advertisements. In fact, in 2004, the agency reviewed only half the number of ads they did in 1999. Some complaints they did not respond to included false or misleading ads and omission of suicide risks.[5]

COUNTERTHINK
"FDA VISION TEST"

As I stated in the Medicine chapter, politicians are taking money from powerful corporations. The top two lobbying industries spent quite a bit of money over a twelve-year period trying to "buy" favorable legislation from politicians:

1. Pharmaceuticals and Health Products: $2,000,000,000

2. Insurance (including health): $1,500,000,000[6]

So what about us? Who is really protecting and representing us? Who is at the helm of this ship? *We are.*

The government and corporations are accountable to voters, taxpayers and consumers. Unfortunately, the public is not paying enough attention to what those in power are doing and so are not holding them accountable. But, who really wants to pay *more* attention to politics and corporations? Boring, right? However, if we want our voices to speak louder than the checks these unethical corporations write, we *have* to get involved.

Many people make excuses like, "It's too complicated" for not paying attention. But, there are people who benefit from the public's lack of interest—people who want power—and they want you to be bored and confused. If you insert yourself into the loop of current events, not only will you be better able to hold those in power accountable, but you will no doubt find it fascinating and sometimes horrifying. Movies like *The Firm* and *Wall Street* are often based on true stories.

The following is an example of this real-life drama. Linda Pino, a former medical insurance reviewer who testified before Congress, admitted to denying a man medical treatment in order to save the company half of a million dollars. This cost the man his life. Pino said she was rewarded, received a good reputation and was promoted for this.[7] There are many stories like this that usually correlate to greed.

The public must spend and vote as informed consumers and constituents. They must do their part to maintain a balance between individuals, industry and government. We, the people, must push on behalf of our own interests just as many corporations and politicians are pushing for theirs.

Chapter Five

Amino Acids

"You are what you eat." – Author unknown

Have you ever heard the saying, "You are what you eat"? Did it mean anything to you? Most people know that foods like doughnuts are bad for you and whole-grain bread is good for you, but do they know why?

Food processing often kills or removes nutrients. A doughnut is more heavily processed than whole grains. During processing, doughnuts have nutrients like amino acids removed. Amino acids comprise our DNA, which is the blueprint for life. It is true that you are what you eat and is especially true when it comes to whole foods and amino acids. Popular nutritional catch phrases must be supported with actual nutrition knowledge to have any real meaning.

I first read about amino acids in *The Vitamin Bible* which details nutrients, like amino acids, and their functions.[1] *The Vitamin Bible* is what first convinced me of the power of nutrition. Amino acids are the foundations of life and were also, ironically enough, the foundation of *my* new life. Reading about amino acids started me on a path that eventually led me to become a nutritionist.

Amino acids are the building blocks of protein. They create energy by turning food into fuel and act as antioxidants, detoxifying our bodies.

Amino acids send messages, catalyze chemical reactions and form molecules such as heme, a component in blood, which transports oxygen and iron and distributes them to the cells of our bodies.

There are approximately 28 commonly known amino acids. 80 percent of amino acids can be made in the body, but the rest cannot, and must be obtained through the diet. The amino acids the body cannot produce are called "essential" amino acids. These include histidine, isoleucine, leucine, lysine, methionine, phenylalanine, threonine, tryptophan and valine. "Non-essential" amino acids include alanine, arginine, asparagine, aspartic acid, citrulline, cysteine, cystine, gamma-amino butyric acid, glutamic acid, glutamine, glycine, ornithine, proline, serine, taurine and tyrosine. Amino acids are found in protein-rich foods like meat, milk, fish, whole grains, beans, nuts and seeds.[2]

When we do not get the right amount of amino acids, our bodies can break down. Imbalances of these nutrients have been implicated in countless health problems, including depression, schizophrenia, ADD, Alzheimer's, autism, dementia, epilepsy, chronic fatigue syndrome, erectile dysfunction, bipolar syndrome, excess body fat, tumor growth and multiple sclerosis.[1, 2,3,4]

Amino acids and other nutrients can be difficult to comprehend, but a basic knowledge of them is essential to understanding nutrition. So scan over this list and the others when you get to them, and try to absorb as much as possible.

Histidine

- Used for tissue repair and nerve cell protection. Removes heavy metals from the system. Lowers blood pressure and may help prevent AIDS.

- Symptoms of imbalance include stress, anxiety, schizophrenia, rheumatoid arthritis and nerve deafness. May aid sexual arousal and sexual functioning. May intensify manic or bipolar symptoms and can contribute to diseases like Alzheimer's, Parkinson's and diabetes.

- Food sources include rice, wheat and rye.[2]

Phenylalanine

- Converted into tyrosine, dopamine and norepinephrine, which promote alertness; interferes with serotonin, which affects mood, sleep and appetite; is a painkiller, antidepressant, and appetite suppressant; aids in memory and learning; can be used to treat arthritis, depression, menstrual cramps, migraines, obesity, Parkinson's disease and schizophrenia.

- Symptoms of imbalance include increased blood pressure, moodiness, and disturbances in sleep and appetite.

- Food sources include beef, chicken, soy, beans, and spirulina or seaweed. It is found naturally in breast milk and in the manufactured food product aspartame. Phenylalanine is added to many foods like sodas and gum.[1, 2]

Taurine

- Maintains eye function; affects blood platelet activity, sperm motility, sperm levels, insulin activity, nervous system function, fat digestion, formation of bile, and heart function; controls cholesterol; has protective effect on the brain, alcohol withdrawal, anxiety, atherosclerosis, congestive heart failure, Down's syndrome, edema, epilepsy, hyperactivity, hypoglycemia, muscular dystrophy, seizures and brain function.

- Symptoms of imbalance include manic episodes, seizures, cardiac arrhythmia and impaired vision.

- Food sources include eggs, fish, meat and milk and many food products like energy drinks.[2, 5, 6]

Tryptophan

- A building block of serotonin, melatonin and niacin; can aid in sleep; is a calming agent and antidepressant; can treat epilepsy and depression; helps with insomnia; stabilizes moods; and is good for migraine headaches and nicotine withdrawal.

- Tryptophan is called the natural alternative to Prozac. Psychiatrists sometimes prescribe tryptophan to those who do not respond to antidepressant drug treatments.

- Symptoms of imbalance include pellagra, coronary artery spasms, depression and insomnia.

- Food sources include brown rice, bananas, milk, yogurt, cottage cheese, red meat, eggs, fish, poultry, mushrooms and corn.[1, 2, 7]

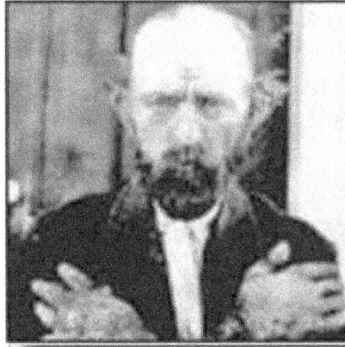

Pellagra

Tyrosine

- A precursor to norepinephrine and dopamine; is a mood elevator and, if deficient, can cause depression; thyroid hormones are derived from tyrosine; contributes to making morphine in the body; can treat medication-resistant depression, anxiety, cocaine and other drug addiction/withdrawal, chronic fatigue syndrome, narcolepsy, low sex drive, allergies, headache and Parkinson's disease.

- Symptoms of imbalance include depression, low blood pressure, low body temperature (cold feet and hands), hypothyroidism and restless leg syndrome.

- Food sources include soy, poultry, fish, almonds, avocados, bananas, milk, cheese, yogurt, lima beans, mushrooms and corn, and is added to many food products including energy drinks.[1,2]

Nutrients and Disease

Pellagra, pictured previously, is a skin disease caused by a tryptophan deficiency. This disease is a good example of the power of nutrients and of man's often confusing search for them. In 1918 a scientist hired to find a cure to the pellagra epidemic that had killed eleven thousand people in the southern U.S. discovered that a high-quality protein diet could cure pellagra. Despite this discovery, pellagra continued to kill.

Pellagra killed more than 27,000 people in the years following the discovery about the relationship between diet and pellagra. The problem was that the B-complex vitamins were not isolated in a lab until 1930. Because scientists did not know tryptophan was a precursor to vitamin B3 they ignored the relationship between diet and pellagra. They simply could not connect the dots.[7]

Many substances and chemical pathways are still yet to be discovered; therefore, we are still missing some dots and, no doubt, still ignoring what works because we haven't isolated all of the reasons in a lab yet.

Nutrients and Synergy

The chemicals in our bodies work together in an intricate balance called "synergy". The word "synergy" is derived from the Greek word "synergos", which means "working together". Amino acids and other nutrients work together and share pathways in our bodies. Nutrients must be in balance or they can be ineffective — either because they have to compete with each other or are missing a necessary counterpart needed to function.

If a weightlifter takes the amino acid arginine to gain muscle mass, for example, his body's ability to absorb another amino acid, lysine, will be reduced. This is because these two amino acids share the same transport systems.[8] This is like two people needing a taxi to get to work but there is only one — and it only has one seat. As a result, only one person at a time can ride. The one left behind *may* find another way to get where they are going, but it won't be as effective.

This taxi analogy can be applied to many nutrients in the body. Imagine all of the potential problems caused by a single nutrient imbalance, which causes a traffic jam on one end and a shortage of nutrients or "workers" on the other. This creates an excess on one side *and* a deficiency on the other. Those nutrients waiting may overfill the waiting area and cause a wall to fall over *and* the jobs on the other end will likely not get done. This can create a chain reaction as even more nutrients have difficulty getting through the clogged area or have trouble working because the nutrients they relied on to do their job didn't show up for work, and so on, to countless other nutrients down the line. This cumulative effect will often cause something along one of the affected chains to break. In the meantime, the body will probably not work as it should, and the host may feel lethargic or sick. The longer an imbalance continues the more likely a break will occur. This describes one of the many ways the body can break after an imbalance and why synergy and balance are so critically important.

By manipulating and adding and removing nutrients like amino acids from foods, food manufacturers are completely ignoring synergy and the fact that nutrients rely on it to work properly.

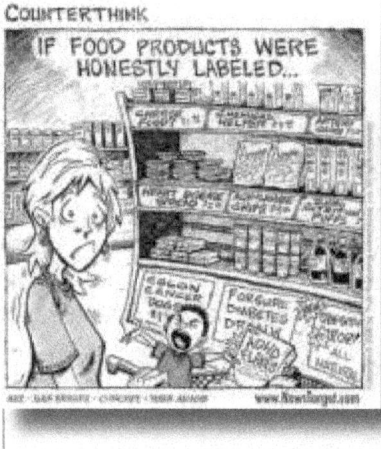

As is the case with energy drinks, diet soda and gum, not only do we add amino acids cavalierly to foods but we also remove them. Many amino acids are removed when making white flour (a primary ingredient in doughnuts, as mentioned earlier), one of the most popular food products on the market today.

The whole wheat grain has three main parts: the bran, germ and endosperm.

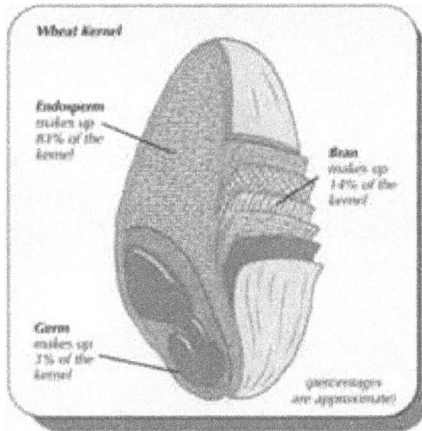

Whole-Wheat Grain

The parts of the whole-wheat grain with the most amino acids are the bran and germ—the parts removed when making white flour. All that is left in white flour is the endosperm, which not only has fewer amino acids, but is full of the protein gluten. Food manufacturers love gluten because it is extremely pliable *and* tasty. Many people are developing gluten allergies as a result of the overconsumption of white flour.

Protein quality depends on all the essential amino acids being present in the right amounts, and in complete proteins they are. According to a measurement by the Institute of Medicine (IOM), a complete protein has a score of 100.[9] Letter grades—based on numeric scores—for the individual parts of the wheat grain are as follows:

Report Card—Wheat Grain	
Grain Component	*Protein Quality*
Germ	A
Bran	C
Endosperm	F

Note: In the Diet chapter, there is more on precisely which nutrients, including amino acids, are removed when processing foods like white flour.

As I said, in order for nutrients like amino acids to do their jobs effectively in the body they must be balanced, and they are in complete proteins and whole foods like whole grains. This explains some of the value of consuming whole foods and knowing which foods to choose.

Too Much of a Good Thing:

The Importance of Balance

Recently some of the many benefits of the soybean were discovered. Soy is a complete protein—rich in amino acids and other nutrients. As a result of these discoveries, many people began to consume large amounts of soy. Soy is being modified and mass-grown and produced. Many people now even take soy supplements. The result? Increasing incidences of soy allergies among the populace. Too much of any substance can cause problems in the body and, if there is one miracle cure, it is balance.

Our society is advanced and has made many beneficial discoveries, but when it comes to our health, Mother Nature still knows best. So until we know more than she knows, we should listen to her wisdom combined with our own and prescribe more whole, organic food—with naturally synergistic amounts of nutrients like amino acids—and balanced diets. If we change course, who knows how many lives could be saved?

Chapter Six

Micronutrients

"The wise man should consider that health is the greatest of human blessings. Let food be your medicine." — Hippocrates

Have you ever heard the statement: "Get your vitamins"?

Micronutrients are nutrients the body needs in small amounts and include vitamins and minerals. The body needs vitamins and minerals to grow, develop, function and heal itself from illness. When our bodies do not get the right amount of any micronutrient, they will not function properly and can break.

We all know we are supposed to eat healthy and get plenty of vitamins and minerals, but we don't know where to find them or *why* we need them, so many of us don't do it.

Vitamins

There are 13 vitamins your body needs that it cannot produce — vitamins A, C, D, E, K and the B vitamins like biotin, niacin, pantothenic acid, riboflavin, thiamine, vitamin B-6, B-9 (folate or folic acid) and B-12. Each vitamin has a specific job.[1]

Vitamin imbalances have been implicated in numerous diseases, including ADD, heart disease, erectile dysfunction, depression, night blindness, skin disorders, chronic fatigue, obesity, diabetes, cholesterol, blood pressure and blood thinness or thickness. Here are the details about some vitamins:

Vitamin A

- Plays an important role in vision, growth, reproduction and immune function.

- Symptoms of imbalance include night blindness, dry eye syndrome, poor growth, dry skin, lowered immunity, headache, vomiting, hair loss, liver damage, skin problems, birth defects and bone pain.

- Food sources include liver, fish, carrots, peaches, leafy greens, sweet potatoes, broccoli and fortified milk.[2]

Vitamin B1/Thiamin

- Enhances circulation; assists in blood formation, carbohydrate metabolism and hydrochloric acid formation (which assists in digestion); optimizes cognitive activity and brain function; has a positive effect on energy, growth, normal appetite and learning capacity; acts as an antioxidant; and contributes to protecting the body from the degenerative effects of aging, alcohol consumption and smoking.

- Symptoms of imbalance include beriberi (a nervous system disease), constipation, edema, enlarged liver, fatigue, forgetfulness, gastrointestinal disturbances, heart changes, irritability, labored breathing, loss of appetite, muscle atrophy, nervousness, numbness of the hands and feet, pain and sensitivity, poor coordination, tingling sensations, weak and sore muscles, general weakness and severe weight loss.

- Food sources include brown rice, eggs, fish, legumes, liver, peanuts, peas, pork, poultry and whole grains.[3]

Vitamin B9/Folic Acid/Folate

- Needed for energy production and formation of red blood cells; aids in formation of white blood cells, therefore strengthening immunity; and participates in DNA and RNA synthesis. Folate helps prevent birth defects and may help treat depression and anxiety.

- Symptoms of imbalance include sore and red tongue, anemia, apathy, digestion disturbances, fatigue, graying hair, growth impairment, insomnia, labored breathing, memory problems, paranoia, weakness and birth defects.

- Food sources include barley, beef, bran, brown rice, cheese, chicken, dates, green leafy vegetables, root vegetables, oranges and whole wheat. Low consumption of fresh fruits and vegetables can cause folic acid deficiencies because cooking kills folic acid.[3]

Vitamin C/Ascorbic Acid

- An antioxidant required for tissue growth and repair, adrenal gland function, and healthy gums; aids in formation of anti-stress hormones; helps metabolize folic acid, tyrosine and phenylalanine; protects against pollution and infection; helps prevent cancer; enhances immunity; increases the absorption of iron; may reduce cholesterol levels and high blood pressure and prevent atherosclerosis; helps with formation of collagen; protects against blood clotting and bruising; and promotes healing of wounds and burns.

- Symptoms of imbalance include scurvy (characterized by poor wound healing), soft and spongy bleeding gums, edema, extreme weakness, hemorrhages under the skin, gums that bleed when brushed, increased susceptibility to infection, joint pains, lack of energy, poor digestion, prolonged healing time, a tendency to bruise easily and tooth loss.

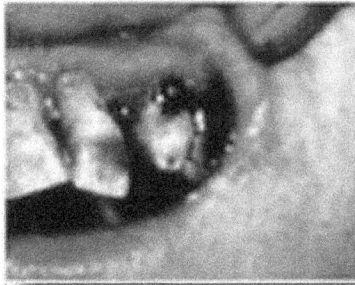

Scurvy

- Food sources include berries, citrus fruits and green vegetables, including asparagus, avocados, oranges, lemons, grapefruit, strawberries, spinach, onions, persimmons, cantaloupe and pineapple.[3]

Vitamin D

- Necessary for the absorption of calcium and phosphorus by the intestinal tract; for growth and for tooth and bone formation; normal blood clotting; thyroid function; regulation of the heartbeat; immunity; and protects against muscle weakness, osteoporosis and hypocalcemia.

- Symptoms of imbalance include rickets, loss of appetite, a burning sensation in the mouth and throat, diarrhea, insomnia, visual problems and weight loss.

- Food sources include fish liver oils, fatty saltwater fish, milk, eggs, butter, tuna, liver, oatmeal and sweet potatoes. Exposure to sunlight is a good source of vitamin D.[3]

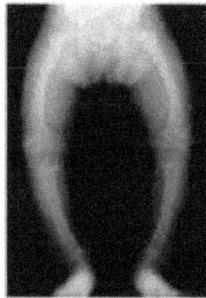
Rickets

Vitamin E

- An antioxidant important in the prevention of cancer and cardiovascular disease; improves circulation; is necessary for tissue repair; useful for treating premenstrual syndrome and fibrocystic disease of the breast; promotes normal blood clotting and healing; reduces scarring; reduces blood pressure; aids in preventing cataracts; improves athletic performance; relaxes leg cramps; maintains healthy nerves, muscles, and capillary walls; promotes healthy skin and hair; helps prevent anemia and an eye disorder called fibroplasia; prevents cell damage; retards aging; protects other fat-soluble vitamins from destruction by oxygen; aids in the body's utilization of vitamin A; and may prevent age spots.

- Symptoms of imbalance include infertility, menstrual problems, destruction of nerves, damage to red blood cells, neuromuscular impairment, shortened red blood cell life span, miscarriage, and uterine degeneration. Deficiencies have been linked to bowel cancer, breast cancer and heart disease.

- Food sources include cold-pressed vegetable oils, dark-green leafy vegetables, legumes, seeds, nuts, brown rice, cornmeal, eggs, kelp, organ meats, oatmeal, soybeans, sweet potatoes, watercress and whole wheat.[3]

Minerals

Minerals come from the earth and are absorbed by plants and water and then by the animals that consume them. The minerals your body needs include calcium, chloride, chromium, copper, fluoride, iodine, iron, magnesium, manganese, molybdenum, phosphorus, potassium, selenium, sodium and zinc. Some minerals, such as lead, are not needed and can be toxic.

Minerals are vital and perform many important functions, like forming bone and skin, and are used for blood flow and oxygen exchange. Mineral imbalances can cause many health problems including autism, depression, fatigue and ADD.[4]

Calcium

- Essential for formation and maintenance of bone and plays a vital role in nerve transmission, muscle contraction, blood pressure regulation and the release of hormones.

- Symptoms of imbalance include loss of bone mass, increased risk of osteoporosis, bone fractures and kidney stones.

- Food sources include milk, cheese, yogurt, sardines, legumes, Chinese cabbage, kale and broccoli.[2]

Fluoride

- Strengthens bones and tooth enamel, eliminates bacteria involved in tooth decay, and can be used to treat osteoporosis and prevent bone fractures.

- Symptoms of imbalance include mottled teeth, tooth decay, kidney damage and abnormal bones. Note: Calcium impairs the absorption of fluoride.

- Food sources include fluoridated water, fish with bones consumed (such as sardines), tea and toothpaste.[2]

Iron

- Aids in producing hemoglobin and is important for enzymes, growth, delivery of oxygen to red blood cells, a healthy immune system and energy production.

- Symptoms of imbalance include anemia, fatigue, decreased resistance to infection, changes in behavior, decreased work capacity, decreased resistance to infection, adverse pregnancy outcomes, inability to adapt to cold weather, pica (desire to eat non-food substances), increased risk of lead poisoning, impaired cognitive ability, weakness and lethargy. Note: Iron works with zinc, copper, manganese and molybdenum and its effectiveness is dependent on the proper balance of each of these nutrients.

- Food sources include red meats, eggs, fish, liver, kidney beans, whole grains, green leafy vegetables and raisins.[2, 3]

Potassium

- Important for a healthy nervous system and regular heart rhythm; helps prevent stroke; aids in proper muscle contraction, water balance and maintaining stable blood pressure; sends electro-chemical impulses; and regulates transfer of nutrients in the body.

- Symptoms of imbalance include dry skin, acne, chills, cognitive impairment, constipation, depression, diarrhea, lowered reflex function, edema, nervousness, thirst, glucose intolerance, irregular heartbeat, insomnia, high cholesterol, low blood pressure, muscular fatigue, headaches, nausea, vomiting, growth impairment, respiratory distress, salt retention and protein in the urine. The function of potassium can decrease with age and this may account for some of the circulatory damage, weakness and lethargy experienced by older people.

- Food sources include dairy foods, fish, fruit, legumes, meat, poultry, vegetables and whole grains.[3]

Sodium

- Necessary for maintaining proper blood pH and water balance and the proper functioning of the stomach, muscles and nerves.

- Symptoms of imbalance include abdominal cramps, anorexia, confusion, dehydration, depression, dizziness, fatigue, flatulence, headache, heart palpitations, lethargy, muscular weakness, memory impairment, poor coordination, recurrent infections, seizures and weight loss. A proper balance of sodium and potassium is necessary in the body. A high intake of sodium can cause a potassium deficiency.

- Virtually all foods contain some sodium, including salt. Most of us get enough and some may get too much, but deficiencies do occur, especially by taking certain medications. More natural sources of sodium are best, including sea salt.[3]

Zinc

- Protects cells from free radical damage; helps heal wounds and is involved in making DNA, breaking down carbohydrates, keeping a balance of acids and bases in the body, immune system function, learning, fertility and sexual performance.

- Symptoms of imbalance include retarded growth, delayed sexual development, loss of appetite, increased infections, dermatitis, hair loss, night blindness, impaired learning and immune system function, gastrointestinal irritation, diarrhea, vomiting, abdominal cramps and headaches. Zinc is commonly deficient in epileptics.[4] Note: Zinc is needed for folate absorption. Phytate can inhibit zinc absorption. Zinc can interfere with copper absorption. Zinc can also be absorbed into certain foods stored in galvanized containers.

- Food sources include red meat, liver, eggs, vegetables, some seafood, whole grains (lost in milling and not replaced like many other nutrients lost in processing) and grain products leavened with yeast.[2]

Some of the illustrations, such as scurvy and rickets, are common in nutrition textbooks and, although they are not prevalent in developed countries, do show the power of nutrients. There *are* many health problems occurring in our populace today as a result of nutrient imbalances, however.

Different foods contain different nutrients. Let's take, for example, some minerals in cheese.

Cheese Type	Calcium (% RDA)	Sodium (Milligrams)
Swiss	52	127
Mozzarella	29	351
Cheddar	48	410

Note: Amounts are based on ½-cup servings.[5] The recommended daily amount for sodium is between 1,500-2,300 milligrams, but most Americans consume 3,400 a day.[6]

Cheddar and mozzarella have more sodium than Swiss cheese, and Swiss and cheddar have more calcium than mozzarella. Deciding which type of cheese to choose could depend on the needs of the individual. So knowledge is power. For instance, would you choose Swiss over cheddar cheese and a heart attack?

Vitamin, mineral and other nutrient imbalances are often at the root of diseases, yet are still being ignored. We already know enough, so doctors, food manufacturers and others who continue to ignore nutrients are being negligent and it must stop.

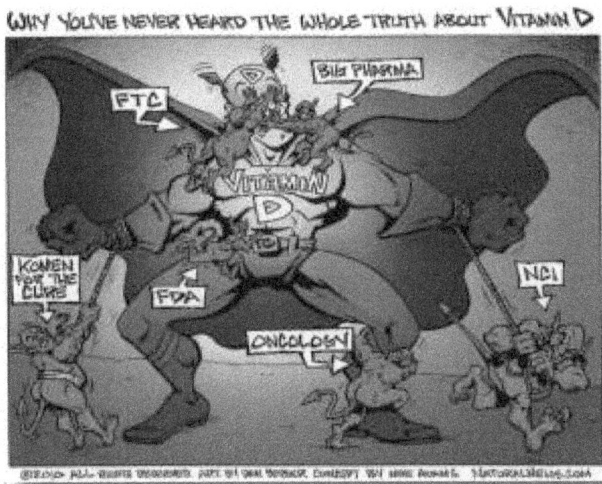

Chapter Seven

Macronutrients

"To eat is a necessity, but to eat intelligently is an art." – *Francois de La Rochefoucauld*

Macronutrients are the nutrients needed by the body in large amounts and include carbohydrates, protein, fat, water and air. As is the case with other nutrients, imbalances of any macronutrient can cause problems in the body.

Carbohydrates

A diet fad of late is a low-carbohydrate, or no-carbohydrate diet. The main problem with that is carbohydrates are the body's primary source of fuel. Carbohydrates are also the only source of energy for the brain and red blood cells. Besides being a major source of energy for the body, carbohydrates have many other health benefits, including having a mild tranquilizing effect. For this reason, carbohydrates can be beneficial for treating seasonal effective disorder and depression. But this may also be why some people over-consume carbs. Again, what we need to achieve with respect to carbohydrates, like all other nutrients, is *balance*.

Carbohydrates come in two forms: simple and complex. They are made up of chains of sugar (glucose) molecules. The longer the chain, the more complex the carbohydrate and the slower it is digested. Simple carbohydrates break down faster and, therefore, cause a quick spike in blood sugar. This quick surge of carbohydrates is hard on the pancreas and other organs. Overconsumption of simple carbs, especially those found in refined foods, can lead to many problems, including hypoglycemia and diabetes. Eating too many simple carbohydrates in processed foods is the problem many people are having these days—not from eating the "good" carbohydrates found in whole foods.

Fiber is an important complex carbohydrate. Fiber is the body's natural cleanser, and helps "clean our pipes" or intestines. Fiber increases turnover of toxins and other waste products by changing the consistency of waste products for a more efficient exit. Clean pipes allow for nutrients to cross through intestinal walls and enter the bloodstream to be used by the body. Not surprisingly, consuming plenty of fiber lowers the risk of colon cancer. Fiber also helps lower blood cholesterol levels and reduces the risk of heart disease. Too much fiber can interfere with nutrient absorption; however, most American diets are lacking in fiber.

Carbohydrates are found almost exclusively in plant foods, with the exception of milk products. Complex carbs are found in plant foods like fruits, vegetables, beans and whole grains. Simple carbs are found in foods like fruit juices, milk, high fructose corn syrup and sugar.[1, 2]

Protein

Proteins are chains of amino acids, as we discussed earlier in the Amino Acid chapter. Proteins make up the greatest portion of our body weight after water and are a part of every living cell. It is needed for growth and development and helps maintain water balance and pH. Proteins make up muscles, ligaments, tendons, organs, glands, hair, nails and vital body fluids. The hormones and enzymes that catalyze and regulate all bodily processes are proteins.[1]

Protein imbalances can cause dehydration, edema, kidney and many other problems, including those listed in the Amino Acid chapter. And kwashiorkor—a disease that occurs in impoverished areas throughout the world—is caused by inadequate levels of protein.

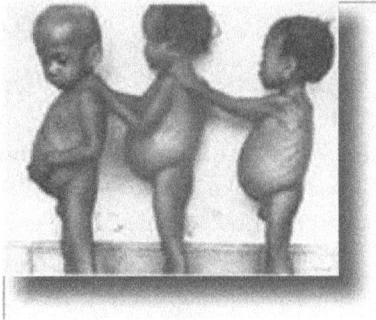

Kwashiorkor

Due to the heavy consumption of animal products in the American diet, most people in the U.S. consume *too much* protein. Animal foods are good sources of protein, but protein can also be found in plant foods. In fact, plant foods lack the saturated fat and cholesterol of animal foods — and have many other nutrients like vitamins, minerals, water and fiber — so plant protein is an excellent choice. As mentioned in the Amino Acid chapter, the amino acids in proteins work together and, if out of balance, will not work as they should; therefore, complete proteins are necessary in the diet. Good sources of complete proteins include eggs, milk, soy, yogurt and rice and bean combinations.

Fat

Most fat is not bad for you as many people believe it is. Your body and brain need fat. Fat performs many important functions: providing insulation for the body and cushion for the organs; protecting against temperature changes; helping with nerve transmission and muscle contraction and being involved in memory.[3]

Too much fat — especially saturated and trans-fats, the so-called "bad" fats — *is* bad for you: causing obesity, heart disease, heart attacks, strokes and more. So-called "good" fats include poly — and mono-unsaturated fats.

Saturated fat is often referred to as the "bad" fat but it is not, in itself, bad for you. The problem is that most of us are consuming too much. Saturated fats are found primarily in animal products like eggs, cheese and meat, but can also be found in plant foods such as coconut and palm kernel oils.

Man-Made Fat

Man-made trans-fat was created in a lab by taking unsaturated fat and attaching hydrogen atoms to it, therefore "saturating" it and making it structurally similar to a "saturated" fat. Both saturated fats and trans-fats are solid at room temperature. Trans-fats are found in many processed foods, including those made with hydrogenated oil. This "test-tube" fat is less healthy than saturated fat.

Olestra is another man-made fat added to foods like potato chips, but, because the fat is not digested properly, it causes problems like anal leakage. We must leave natural substances like fat alone, and instead just try to eat them in the right amounts.

Cholesterol

Cholesterol is important for cell structure, digestion, absorption and making hormones.[3] Cholesterol is considered by many in the public to be unhealthy. But again, the actual problem is that most people are consuming too much. The human body can make its own cholesterol. Cholesterol is found in animal products like eggs, butter, meat and shellfish.

Digging Deeper into Fatty Foods

One of the fatty foods that get a bad rap — but which is actually good for you — is the avocado. Avocadoes are rich in the "good" or unsaturated fat *and* fat-soluble vitamins that need fat to be absorbed and utilized by the body. The avocado is a great example of the natural synergy contained in whole foods.

Some people think all cheese is bad for you. This is not true. For example, let's compare saturated fat and cholesterol content of cheddar, Swiss and mozzarella cheese.

Cheese Type	Saturated Fat (Grams)	Cholesterol (Milligrams)
Cheddar	14	70
Swiss	12	61
Mozzarella	8	44

Note: Amounts are based on ½-cup servings.[4] The daily limit for cholesterol is less than 200 or 300 milligrams a day (depending on risk level). However, most men eat about 350 and women about 240 milligrams a day. The daily limit for saturated fat is 7-10% (14-20 grams for a 2,000-calorie-per-day diet) of total calories, which most Americans also exceed.[5]

An all-too-easy answer for a healthy diet is to avoid cheese and other fatty foods altogether. But cheese, and many other foods thought to be unhealthy, *can* be a part of a healthy, balanced diet. The answer is education, not avoidance.

Water

Elizabeth's Healthy Spritzer
Ingredients:
4 ounces 100% fruit juice
4 ounces carbonated water
½ cup ice
Directions: Pour all ingredients into glass and enjoy!

Many people don't understand why they should drink water, and, when a drink like this is proposed to them, just think, "That's one more thing I need to do, and I *love* my soda!" Without knowledge about what water (and soda, for that matter) does for your body, there is not enough motivation to change. But once you learn about *why* you should drink water, there is more desire for a drink like *Elizabeth's Healthy Spritzer*.

Water provides a place for chemical reactions to occur; participates in many chemical reactions; regulates body temperature; removes waste products; transports nutrients; maintains acid-base balance and processes vitamins. Water affects everything in the body. Imbalances can, therefore, cause a malfunction of just about any bodily function. Symptoms of water imbalance include excess body fat, poor muscle tone, digestive problems, poor functioning of organs — including the brain — muscle soreness and water retention.

Water can help alleviate many health problems, including stomachaches, headaches and fatigue. Water can slow the aging process, lessen the intensity and number of incidences of arthritis, and help alleviate kidney stones, digestion problems, constipation, obesity, diabetes and glaucoma.

Unfortunately, water can be unhealthy *and* unsafe. Many water companies do not meet the basic requirements of the Environmental Protection Agency (EPA) for safe levels of toxic substances. Some of these include arsenic, copper, iron, radon, lead, fluoride and other heavy metals.[1, 3]

Air

Air is a nutrient critical to life. Humans and plants have a symbiotic relationship, as we literally feed each other. We breathe in oxygen (O_2) and breathe out carbon dioxide (CO_2). Plants breathe out O_2 and breathe in CO_2. Oxygen is the most powerful substance in the body and has the ability to provide life to all of its cells.

Not all air is good for you. A 2010 American Lung Association "State of the Air" report found that roughly 58 percent of the population suffers pollution levels that are often too dangerous to breathe. Over time, exposure to these particles, mainly from factories and cars, may increase the risk of asthma, lung damage and death.[6]

Toxins are present in our air, water and food and most people don't consume enough of the foods — mainly plant foods — that help rid the body of these harmful substances. Therefore, we must fully investigate the effects toxins have on our health — and, of course, eat more of the healthy foods that help eliminate these dangerous chemicals from the body.

There is a lot to cover when it comes to nutrition, and this book is not designed to cover every nutrient in detail, but it is designed to give you enough information to illustrate the fundamentals of nutrition.

Chapter Eight

Diet

"A vegetarian manner of living . . . would most beneficially influence the lot of mankind." — Albert Einstein

"Eat healthy."

"Eat a balanced diet."

Has the doctor made either of these suggestions to you? Do you know what these statements mean? Do they mean sugar-free, fat-free, no carbohydrate, Jenny Craig, Weight Watchers, South Beach, Atkins diet food or Slim-Fast shakes? Do you think they mean eating salad with no dressing, no fried food, no fast food, no junk food and no dessert?

Healthy eating means eating foods with nutrients your body needs to function. It means eating the "bad" stuff, but not all of the time. Food can give you energy and heal you. Healthy eating can be fun and satisfying. We need to *eat* food, not avoid it. We must change our philosophy about food, and our approach to diet, but first we must understand nutrition.

Calorie Counting

Many people are familiar with the term "calories". Many dietitians say, "A calorie is a calorie." This implies that all you need to concern yourself within your diet is the number of calories you consume. A calorie is an accurate form of energy measurement, but it is virtually useless as a form of nutrient measurement. Many people are concerned with losing weight and this has been a simple approach needed for busy lives, but it isn't enough.

The calorie-counting approach is simple — too simple — and this oversimplification is why calorie-counting alone often doesn't work. For instance, many people avoid fat because it is high in calories. Fat does contain more calories than carbohydrates or protein do, but fat is also very satisfying (more dense and so you need less to become full). Plus, we need fat. Fat, like all other nutrients, just needs to be kept in balance in the diet.

When I received my nutrition education, no one said to me, "A calorie is a calorie. Now go count the calories for all your patients." If all that mattered were calories, I would have been better off with a math and not a pre-med degree.

Counting calories is like saying all that matters in a game—for instance, a professional basketball game—is the final score. If that were true, you could just skip the game and check the final score every day. It is the same in basketball as it is in the body: it is also *how* the points were scored that matter.

A vacuum of missing nutrition information in our society has created a need for short answers, hence the calorie-counting obsession. If calorie-counting was all we needed to worry about then we could all eat doughnuts all the time and be as healthy as someone who eats carrots all the time. There are vast differences in the nutrients contained within these foods. The question, then, is *how* to get the proper amount of calories. The answer is through a balanced diet.

The idea behind calorie counting is that successful calorie counters will consume more nutrient-dense foods like fruits and vegetables, which have fewer calories than many unhealthy foods. This is a good theory; if it worked it would be even better.

The 80/20 Formula

I came up with a simple plan for healthy eating after years of intensive study, which I call the 80/20 formula. The 80/20 method is popular because most people want simple rules they can follow and do not want to be deprived of their favorite things. With this formula, they don't have to.

The 80/20 formula means bending the rules 20 percent of the time and doing what is right for the rest. For example, one soda per day would be close to consuming 20 percent of the foods we should limit, or "bad" foods, allowed for the day and the rest of the day would need to be spent eating nutritiously.

Most of us are not getting the nutrients our bodies need because of our unbalanced diets. A standard American fast food meal is a McDonald's meal—a burger, fries and soda—which is roughly 1,400 calories.[1] Assuming you had a daily caloric requirement of 2,000 calories, eating just two of these meals a day already puts you over your daily limit by 800 calories. This meal is also high in saturated fat, sugar, salt and cholesterol—all the "bad" stuff that causes obesity, diabetes and hypertension.

If you were to consume a McDonald's meal or other fatty, highly processed, unhealthy meal, as part of the 80/20 program, you could do it successfully.
Unfortunately, most people have the 80/20 in reverse and don't know it.

The US Department of Agriculture Food Guides

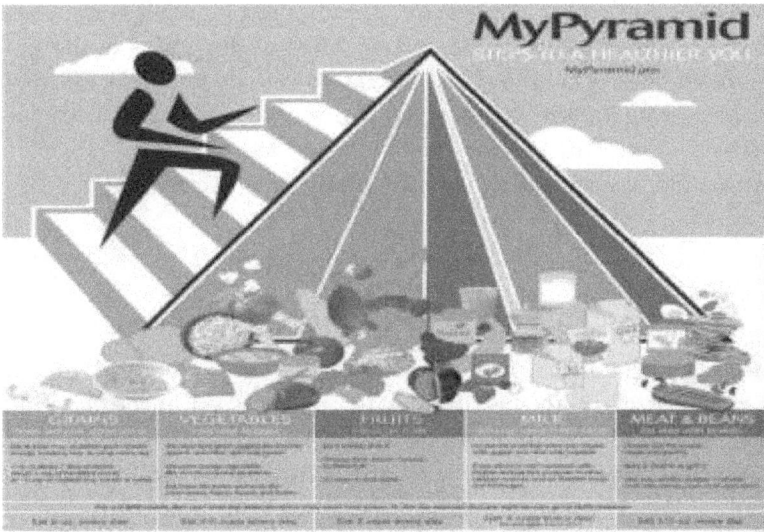

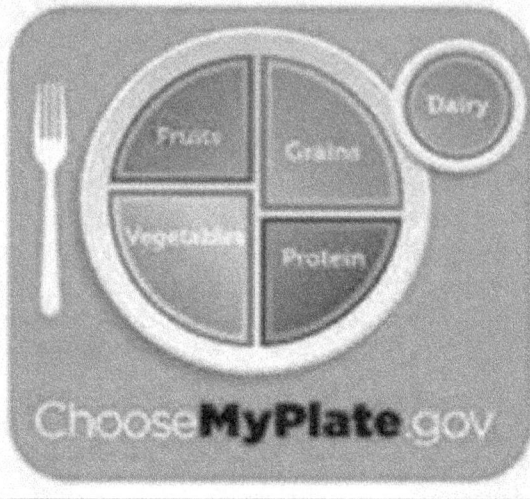

The USDA's food guide, which used to be a pyramid, but is now a plate, is another oversimplification of the complex nature of nutrition, but can be a useful guide.

The first part of the pyramid/plate—where you find grains, vegetables and fruits—is where you should find the bulk of your nutrients, and most people don't. Our choices are often limited by what is most readily available in our markets. Need grains? Most of the grains in the grocery store are in the form of sugary breakfast cereals and processed white flour. Need vegetables? Most of us are relying on french fries for our vegetables. Our fruits are mostly ingested in juice form. And unfortunately, we are eating way too many processed foods.

Processed Food

Whole, raw food is naturally rich in many nutrients, and processing them removes many of their nutrients, as discussed in the Amino Acid chapter. Scientists are still learning about the many nutrients in foods so, oftentimes, we don't even know what we are destroying.

We heat food for taste and to kill dangerous pathogens. However, heat also destroys *nutrients,* because the bonds that hold them together are broken and they die. Cooking can cause a nutrient loss of up to 80 percent in vegetables. It is what is being destroyed along with the pathogens that should also give us concern.

Let's look at the nutrients lost by processing whole apples into applesauce and juice.

Nutrient	Units	Whole Apple	Applesauce	Apple Juice
Macronutrient				
Fiber	G	3	2	0
Sugars	G	14	23	13
Minerals				
Beta Carotene	Mcg	37	0	0
Choline	Mg	5	0	3
Fluoride	Mcg	5	0	0
Folate	Mcg	4	1	0
Lutein	Mcg	40	0	22
Magnesium	Mg	7	4	7
Phosphorus	Mg	15	10	10
Potassium	Mg	148	84	139
Sodium	Mg	1	39	6
Vitamins				
Vitamin A	IU	75	15	1
	RAE, Mcg	4	1	0
Vitamin C	Mg	6	2	1
Vitamin K	Mcg	3	0	0

Amounts are based on the size of a medium apple (138 grams).[1]

Whole apples have more nutrients than applesauce or juice. Nutrients are lost during each step of processing. Processing apples into sauce causes nutrient losses; further processing into juice causes even more.

As discussed in the Amino Acid chapter, white flour, the most common flour on the market, contains one part of the grain, the endosperm — the part with the least nutritional value. Let's compare the nutritional differences between white flour and whole-wheat flour.

Nutrient	Units	Whole-Wheat Flour	White Flour
Macronutrient			
Energy	kCal	407	455
Protein	G	16.44	12.91
Carbohydrate	G	87.08	95.39
Fiber	G	14.6	3.4
Minerals			
Calcium	Mg	41	19
Iron	Mg	4.66	1.46
Magnesium	Mg	166	28
Phosphorus	Mg	415	135
Potassium	Mg	486	134
Sodium	Mg	6	2
Zinc	Mg	3.52	0.88
Copper	Mg	0.458	0.180
Manganese	Mg	4.559	0.853
Selenium	Mcg	84.8	42.4
Vitamins			
Thiamin	Mg	0.536	0.150
Riboflavin	Mg	0.258	0.050

Niacin	Mg	7.638	1.562
Pantothenic acid	Mg	1.210	0.547
Vitamin B-6	Mg	0.409	0.055
Folate	Mcg	53	32
Choline	Mg	37.4	13.0
Betaine	Mg	87.4	0.0
Carotene, beta	Mcg	6	0
Vitamin A, IU	IU	11	0
Lutein + zeaxanthin	Mcg	264	22
Vitamin E (alphatocopherol)	Mg	0.98	0.07
Vitamin K (phylloquinone)	Mcg	2.3	0.4
Fats			
Fatty acids, saturated	G	0.386	0.194
Fatty acids, monounsaturated	G	0.278	0.109
Fatty acids, polyunsaturated	G	0.935	0.516
Amino acids			
Tryptophan	G	0.254	0.159
Threonine	G	0.474	0.351
Isoleucine	G	0.610	0.446
Leucine	G	1.111	0.887
Lysine	G	0.454	0.285
Methionine	G	0.254	0.229
Cystine	G	0.380	0.274

Phenylalanine	G	0.775	0.650
Tyrosine	G	0.480	0.390
Valine	G	0.742	0.519
Arginine	G	0.770	0.521
Histidine	G	0.380	0.287
Alanine	G	0.584	0.415
Aspartic acid	G	0.844	0.544
Glutamic acid	G	5.190	4.349
Glycine	G	0.662	0.464
Proline	G	1.706	1.498
Serine	G	0.775	0.645

Amounts are based on 1-cup serving.[1]

As you can see from this list, whole-wheat flour has many more nutrients than white flour. Notice, also, that the list is much longer than on standard food labels. Our bodies need all of these nutrients and so we should consider them all.

Did you know that food makers try to make their food addicting? A phrase on one popular potato chip commercial says, "You can't eat just one." This is not an accident; they actually work at it. Don't believe it? Take white flour, for instance. White flour contains less of the nutrients that help you feel full, like fiber and protein, so many people eat more of the products made with white flour in an attempt to feel satisfied.

The problem with consuming too much processed food is that it does not have nutrients our bodies need, often only makes us hungrier and regularly has dangerous chemicals added to it. This has created a perpetual snowball of failure and our bodies will continue to break if it doesn't stop.

Plant-Based Diets

Study after study shows that consumption of fruits and vegetables and other plant foods correlates to lower incidence of almost all diseases; still, most of us don't eat enough.

It *is* possible to survive off of plant food alone. People who do are called "vegans". Vegans do not consume *any* animal products. "Vegetarians" consume some animal products, like eggs, milk and cheese. The difficulty faced by both vegetarians and vegans — and carnivores too, for that matter — is getting the right amount of nutrients. Plant-based diets often require eating more food than carnivorous ones. People who choose to be vegans or vegetarians mainly do so for health, moral or environmental reasons.

Plant-based diets are often very healthy; however, it is possible to consume animal products and still be healthy. But, since the majority of people need to eat more plant foods, most, therefore, should probably become more "vegan".

Meal Planning

Here is a sample menu that follows the 80/20 formula and USDA food guide:

Day One

Breakfast

1 cup whole-grain cereal or oatmeal with honey* to taste

1/2 peach

1-2 cups water, *Elizabeth's Healthy Spritzer*, coffee or tea

Snack

3/4 cup cottage cheese with fruit

<u>Lunch</u>

1 tuna salad sandwich on whole-grain bread with tomatoes, lettuce and 2 tsp. of regular mayonnaise* or plain yogurt

1 serving Sunchips, baked or regular chips*

1 cup water, herbal tea or *Elizabeth's Healthy Spritzer*

1 apple

<u>Snack</u>

1-2 stalks celery with cream cheese* or peanut butter or 8-10 baby carrot sticks w/ranch dressing*

<u>Dinner</u>

1 chicken breast sautéed in olive or canola oil and fresh herbs

1 cup roasted red potatoes with olive or canola oil, salt* and pepper

1 cup sautéed or baked asparagus with olive oil and lemon pepper

<u>Dessert</u>

3/4 cup ice cream* or 1-2 cookies*

Day Two

<u>Breakfast</u>

1 egg*

1 piece of whole-grain toast with canola oil margarine

1 banana

1 cup coffee, tea or *Elizabeth's Healthy Spritzer*

Snack

1/2 cup plain or vanilla* yogurt with fresh or frozen blueberries and honey* to taste (for plain yogurt)

Lunch

1 cup whole-grain pasta with marinara sauce or 2 slices pizza*

1 cup romaine lettuce, Caesar salad dressing*, croutons*, parmesan cheese

1-2 cups water flavored with lemon or *Elizabeth's Healthy Spritzer*

Snack

3/4 cup almonds or trail mix

Dinner

1 eggplant or steak* with lobster tail* or shrimp* and vegetables and potato, brown or white* rice

1-2 pieces of white* or whole-wheat bread with olive oil, butter* or margarine*

1-2 drinks of choice (water, juice*, soda*, milk*, wine*, beer* or *Elizabeth's Healthy Spritzer*)

Dessert

3/4 cup frozen yogurt* or other low-fat dessert*

Note: This menu was created for a moderately active, adult female. Serving sizes vary depending on gender, age, weight, etc. Items with an asterisk (*) are in the "bad" column for various reasons, such as sugar, saturated or trans-fat, cholesterol, salt, white flour or preservative content. Of course, each individual can choose their own "bad" foods.

"Day Two" has the option for steak, lobster or shrimp, eggs and butter. These foods are all high in cholesterol. Because this menu includes these foods, the next day would not be a good day for more high-cholesterol foods. Instead, lean protein sources and lots of fruits and vegetables would be great choices.

A balanced diet can still contain all of the things you like, and many people like pizza. Many are surprised to learn they can still eat pizza and be healthy. A healthy way to eat pizza is by eating a thin or whole-grain crust and loading up on vegetables or lean meats and adding a side salad. The salad helps create a more balanced meal and takes the place of another slice of pizza. You can eat regular crust, you can even order pepperoni, but you wouldn't want to get carried away with white flour or saturated fat for the rest of the day or week. The key, again, is balance.

You may have expected only to see foods like plain carrots or celery sticks, as that is what you are accustomed to seeing from a "dietitian". But we must be realistic to succeed. With the 80/20 formula you can eat just about whatever you want, as long as the "bad" food is less than 20 percent of your overall intake and the rest of your diet is healthy. Healthy means a whole, organic, fresh (raw, whenever possible), balanced diet that follows the USDA food guide. This ratio plan is more realistic than trying not to eat butter or ice cream ever again.

Diets typically don't work because they focus on surface changes based on minimal information. Most diets involve deprivation and will power and so weight loss is usually temporary. The key to a successful "diet" is understanding nutrition on a deep level to create lasting lifestyle changes.

Learning about nutrition and thinking about food from a positive standpoint and focusing on what to eat—instead of what *not* to eat— creates choices, not restriction. And, after learning how to eat, one becomes almost addicted and *wants* to eat healthy because an optimally functioning body feels good.

A nutrition education is far superior to yo-yo dieting, but, of course, if you'd rather, you can continue to try each new diet fad, hoping the next one will be "the one".

Chapter Nine

Research

"Problems cannot be solved at the same level of awareness that created them." –
Albert Einstein

One must make the argument for change in our society's philosophy about nutrition armed with information. Some of the arguments you will hear against it are: "Nutrition is quackery," "Nutrition is unproven," "You need these pills or you might die," "We can't afford to change," "It is impossible," and "We can't do it."

The answers to those arguments are that there *is* a lot of research out there, so it is not unproven. We *can* do it; the research shows that. We *can* afford it, because we spend a lot of money now on failure. We can, instead, save this money and redirect it toward effective solutions — the research also proves *that*. And, we don't *need* medications that only treat symptoms and cause other health problems. Our current path is unsustainable. So not only *can* we do it, we *must* do it.

Even though data exists proving nutrition works, we do need more. But, who will fund it? Apple farmers? Spinach farmers? The problem is, as I mentioned in the Medicine chapter, there is not very much money in apples or spinach and those whose motivation is to make money, like drug manufacturers, are funding most health research today. There is now a disparity between research for profitable solutions and less-profitable solutions — like drugs vs. nutrition.

The Scientific Method

Scientific research is based upon the scientific method. In nutrition, the scientific method offers a systematic, unbiased approach to evaluating the relationships between food, nutrients and health.

The first step of the scientific method is to make an observation and ask questions about it. Then, an explanation is proposed, called a "hypothesis".

Experiments are then performed to test this hypothesis. Critical in this process is the next point: these experiments *must* provide objective results that can be measured and *repeated*.

Next, a theory can be developed. A theory is an explanation based on a compilation of many experiments and repeated results. If most of the results do not prove the original hypothesis wrong, a theory is established. A theory must be continually supported by new, sound evidence for it to remain in place as the best known answer to a hypothesis.

A well designed study is one of the main keys to success in science and to finding the true answer to a question. There is no room for personal opinions in scientific research except to form a hypothesis and comment on conclusions — and then, only after data is collected and recorded. The data must be allowed to speak in an uninhibited manner.

Ideally, study results are interpreted in a peer-review system to account for any investigator bias.[1] In science, bias can still occur, but the system is designed to prevent it as much as possible.

If you follow the scientific method, science should rarely be controversial. We should also be cautious when any one study finds new results, because these experiments must be repeated. The scientific method, in short, is a way to answer a question to the best of human beings' ability.

As I mentioned, a lot of today's research is being funded by financially interested parties. Researchers often feel pressure to find an outcome that pleases the funder. This has affected study results.[2, 3] If there is bias in research, the scientific method simply will not work.

Research Studies

Here are several research studies that illustrate the power of nutrition and support many of the arguments presented in this book.

Attention Deficit Disorder (ADD)

- Study results have shown that artificial food coloring and benzoate preservatives have a negative effect on the behavior of children.[4]

- Fifty-nine of 78 children with hyperactive behavior placed on an elimination diet had improved behavior.[5]

- Study results have shown 3 percent of gifted children had borderline hypoglycemic conditions and allergies. When combined with sensitivity and intensity, this leads to behavior that mimics ADD symptoms.[6]

- Foods and additives are common causes of ADD in children. In one study, almost 75 percent had an adverse reaction. These children reacted to many foods, dyes, and preservatives. Results demonstrated a beneficial effect of eliminating reactive foods and artificial colors in children with ADD. The researchers concluded that dietary factors may play a significant role in the etiology of the majority of children with ADD.[7]

- Scientists conducted a randomized six-week, double-blind, placebo-controlled trial of 44 outpatient children who had been diagnosed with ADD. The study was conducted in order to see if using the mineral zinc in addition to methylphenidate or Ritalin could alleviate the symptoms of ADD more than drugs alone. There have been other studies that have found zinc alone helps reduce ADD symptoms. Zinc plays a role in regulating the brain chemicals melatonin and dopamine. Melatonin affects sleep patterns. Dopamine affects many things, including attention. All of the children in the study had been clearly diagnosed with ADD.

The results of this study showed a reduction in ADD symptoms in both groups of children. At six weeks, the improvement in the group supplemented with zinc was greater than that of the placebo. The improvement seen in the behavior of both groups was similar, but significant improvement was seen and reported on the Teacher Parent Rating Scale in the group supplemented with zinc. This study substantiates the hypothesis that there is a relationship between zinc and ADD symptoms.[8]

• A clinical trial was performed on children ages eight and ten who were found to be iron deficient. Iron deposits are found in areas of the brain where dopamine is regulated. Dopamine levels affect concentration and attention. It was hypothesized that iron deficiencies might lead to imbalances of dopamine, which, in turn, would lead to attention deficits. The results of the study showed a significant improvement in the test scores of iron-deficient children after iron supplementation. These results show a strong correlation between attention and iron deficiency.[9]

Bipolar Disorder

• Supplements of omega-3 fatty acids can have a positive effect on bipolar disorder. In one such study, omega-3 helped stabilize the condition of patients with this disorder. A different dose lowered patients' aggression.[10]

Depression

• Study results have shown that tyrosine, phenylalanine and tryptophan all affect depression.[11]

Eating Disorders

• In a study published in the *Archives of General Psychiatry,* those with a history of bulimia nervosa given an amino acid supplement without tryptophan experienced a relapse more often than those who were given a balanced amino acid supplement.[12]

Cognition and Memory

- Low blood levels of vitamin D may be associated with increased odds of cognitive impairment.[13]

- Study results have shown that a vitamin C deficiency in the first weeks of life results in impaired neuronal development and a decrease in memory in guinea pigs.[14]

Schizophrenia

- Consumption of refined sugar results in a decreased state of mind for schizophrenic patients. Diet may be able to predict schizophrenia and depression.

- A Danish study showed that better prognoses for schizophrenic patients strongly correlate with living in a country where there is a high consumption of omega-3 fatty acids. The omegas have been shown to help depressive patients and can also be used to treat schizophrenia. Furthermore, supplements taken on a daily basis help healthy individuals and schizophrenic patients maintain a balanced mood and improved blood circulation.

- Schizophrenic patients have been found to have an impaired ability to make serotonin, which can come from amino acids. High doses of glycine have been shown to reduce some symptoms of schizophrenia—such as social withdrawal, emotional flatness, and apathy—that don't respond to today's medications. A 1996 clinical trial revealed that glycine could be given to schizophrenic patients without producing adverse side effects.[15]

Weight Loss

- African mango supplementation resulted in one study's participants losing an average of 28 pounds each. The participants also had lowered cholesterol and blood sugar. Participants who did not take the supplement had no notable weight loss. Earlier studies also found this result.[16]

Asthma and Allergies

- Research findings suggest links between folate and allergies and asthma. In a study funded by the National Institutes of Health, researchers reviewed medical data from 8,083 patients from a 2005-2006 study where serum folate levels and the levels of antibodies present in allergic reactions were measured. Higher levels of folate were linked to lower antibody levels, fewer reports of allergies, less wheezing and a lower likelihood of developing asthma. Lower levels of folate were related to a 40 percent increase in the likelihood of an attack. The researchers concluded that additional research was needed to confirm these early findings and to understand the mechanisms involved.[17]

- Study results showed a reduced risk of asthma by 50 percent in children who increased their intake of whole grains and fish.[18]

Blood

- There may be links between vitamin C and blood pressure. In one study, researchers concluded that those with the highest levels of vitamin C had the lowest blood pressure.[19]

- Study results have shown that green and brown algae have strong anticoagulant or blood-thinning activity, suggesting possible potential for the treatment of blood clots.[20]

- Many nutrients have good scientific evidence for treating high blood pressure, including omega-3 fatty acids, fish oil, alpha-linolenic acid, hibiscus, stevia, calcium and Coenzyme Q10.[21]

Bone Density

- Researchers discovered that genistein, a nutrient found in soybeans and peanuts, may help increase bone health by reducing bone loss in women with low bone density. One such study concluded that genistein has positive effects on bone mineral density.

- Other nutritional therapies with strong, good or notable preliminary evidence in the treatment of low bone density include calcium, vitamin D, black tea, boron, copper, creatine, dehydroepiandrosterone (DHEA), gamma linolenic acid, horsetail, red clover, soy, tamarind and vitamin K.[22]

Cancer

- Study results have shown that citrus components tangeretin and nobiletin can stop cancerous cell growth and significantly suppress cancer cell proliferation. Based on these results, it has been determined that citrus may be an effective anticancer agent.[23]

- Mushrooms are now being considered in cancer treatment for their effects on cancer cells, including their anti-tumor effects.[24,25]

- A long-term study was done on 48 men age 60 and up who underwent treatment for prostate cancer. All of the men had rising prostate specific antigen (PSA) levels after treatment. Increased PSA levels are associated with prostate cancer. During the six-year follow-up, men who drank pomegranate juice had lower PSA levels than those who had stopped drinking the juice. At the end of the study, it took four times longer for their PSA levels to double than it had at the beginning of the study.[26]

- Study results have shown consumption of polyphenon E, an ingredient in green tea, led to cancer regression and tumor reduction in significant numbers of patients—over 50 percent of participants in one study.[27]

Fruit and Vegetable Consumption

- Only 26 percent of adults in the U.S. eat vegetables three or more times a day.[28] The following image is from one of my UC-Davis clinical nutrition courses. This table, once deciphered, illustrates a close relationship between consuming fruits and vegetables and a lower risk of all types of cancer. For example, in lung cancer, 24 out of 25 studies showed a correlation between consumption of fruits and vegetables and reduced risk of lung cancer.

Epidemiologic Studies of Fruit and Vegetable Intake and Cancer Risk

Cancer Site	Number of Studies (Protective)	Inverse Association
		(P<0.05)
All Sites, except prostate	156	128
Stomach	19	17
Colorectal	27	20
Bladder	5	3
Cervix	8	7
Ovary	4	3
Breast	14	8
Prostate	14	4
Lung	25	24
Larynx	4	4
Oral Cavity, Pharynx	9	9
Esophagus	16	15
Pancreas	11	9

- There was a similar graph that showed how meat consumption *increased* cancer risk.[29]

Magical Mushrooms

- Mushrooms have many medicinal powers and are considered to be the most powerful food in Chinese medicine. Mushrooms are good for your brain and nervous system and also for your skin and hair. They can enhance immunity; lower blood sugar levels, cholesterol and blood pressure; aid respiration; may cure skin rashes; are anti-inflammatory, anti-bacterial, anti-tumor and anti-viral; and are good for anti-aging.[24] Mushrooms are also used in cancer treatment as described in Cancer above.

Nutrition and Learning

- Children who participated in the Universal School Breakfast Program performed better in school. These children who were at nutritional risk had an increase in grades and decrease in attendance and behavior problems. Participation in a school breakfast program enhanced daily nutrient intake. Improvement in nutrient intake was associated with significant improvement in math grades and behavior in children who were not at nutritional risk.[30]

The Power of Suggestion

- A 2007 Yale University study found that only 40 percent of students regularly ate fruit with their meal, but, when it was offered to them, 70 percent of them did.[31]

Nutrition Education

- A study done by the USDA found that 69 percent of participants in a nutrition education program had an increase in nutrition knowledge and 61 percent had an increased ability to select low-cost, nutritious foods. The entire group showed an overall improvement in their consumption of fruits and vegetables. Adults in the same program showed a 91 percent improvement in consumption of nutritious foods and 88 percent improved their nutrition practices.

- At the start, only 20 percent had reported consuming at least 50 percent of the daily recommended amount of fruits and vegetables. At the end, this increased to 41 percent. The researchers concluded there were a limited number of educational opportunities and resources for nutrition education.[32]

- School garden program participants increased their consumption of fruits and vegetables. Students who participated in a Berkeley, CA, school garden program ate 1.5 servings more fruits and vegetables a day than those who did not participate in the program.[28]

Research Conflict of Interest

- The *American Journal of Psychiatry* took an in-depth look at financial conflict of interest in clinical trials — research that, it is believed, had never been done before — and found a greater likelihood of reporting results favorable to the source of the funding. The researchers examined the funding source and author financial conflict of interest in all clinical trials published in psychiatry journals between 2001 and 2003. They found that, of 397 clinical trials studied, 239 (60 percent) reported receiving funding from a pharmaceutical company or other interested party. 187 studies (50 percent) included at least one author with a reported financial conflict of interest.

- Among the 162 studies examined, those that reported conflict of interest were about five times more likely to report positive results among the pharmaceutical industry-funded studies. The researchers concluded that author conflict of interest was prevalent in psychiatric clinical trials and led to "a greater likelihood of reporting a drug to be superior to placebo."[3]

Medical School Nutrition Education

- Ninety-nine of 106 accredited U.S. medical schools surveyed required some form of nutrition education; however, only 32 schools required a separate nutrition course. On average, students received only 24 hours of nutrition instruction.

- Only 40 medical schools required the minimum recommended by the National Academy of Sciences, which is 25 hours.

- Approximately 90 percent of instructors expressed the need for additional nutrition instruction.[33]

Healthcare Cost Savings

- According to a report by the National Academy of Sciences Institute of Medicine (IOM), getting nutritional therapy is cost effective. Dietitians can help people manage conditions such as high blood pressure, high cholesterol, diabetes and kidney and heart problems. In a study done by the Department of Veterans Affairs, more than half of the people who saw a dietitian lowered their cholesterol and no longer needed cholesterol medication. Nutrition therapy ended up saving the healthcare system $60,000 per year in prescription drug costs.

- On a national level, according to the IOM report, such savings can translate into millions. If Medicare beneficiaries with high blood pressure received nutrition therapy, healthcare costs over a five-year period could be cut by an estimated $52 million to $167 million for hypertension alone. Findings like this led the IOM report's authors to conclude that Medicare should cover physician-ordered nutrition counseling.[34]

There *is* evidence proving nutrition works, yet it is largely being ignored. We do need more research, but we also need funding for it. In the meantime, we should listen to *existing* research. If we do not start to focus more on remedies like nutrition it will not be because the data didn't exist — but because we chose to ignore it.

We should use the scientific method more, and, as it was designed, to answer questions and solve problems. Let's find what works!

Chapter Ten

The Brain

"It's bizarre that the produce manager is more important to my children's health than the pediatrician." — Meryl Streep

Nutrition affects our bodies and our brains. Four of the ten leading causes of disability in developed countries, including the U.S., are mental disorders. There has been an increase in the number of mental health disorders in developed countries due to the deterioration of the Western diet.[1]

Many nutrients have been found to be deficient in patients suffering from mental disorders. But, very few mentally ill patients are treated naturally and are instead given powerful medications. These drugs often cause severe side effects, including dulled personality, reduced emotions, memory loss and tremors.[1, 2]

Nutrition has been found to play a role in addiction, anxiety, attention deficit disorder (ADD), autism, bipolar disease, dementia, depression, eating disorders, obsessive compulsive disorder, schizophrenia and many other mental disorders.[1, 3]

Many nutritional studies were being done in the 70s and 80s on how nutrition may play a role in disorders of the brain, but much of the research was dropped due to underfunding.[1]

ADD

ADD is a subject close to my heart as I was inspired by children suffering from ADD to go back to school and study nutrition. The many children suffering from this disorder also inspired me to get up, out of my warm bed and to biochemistry class on some cold and early mornings.

Because of our rushed society, kids today are eating more junk food, more poor-quality food and more food on the go than any other generation in this country's history. Their educations suffer, too. Children cannot focus, pay attention or learn because their bodies are chemically out of balance. It is heart-wrenching to consider all that diet-induced imbalances are doing to children's small, growing bodies.

ADD is a name given to a set of symptoms with no known cause, though emerging scientific evidence suggests it relates to chemical imbalances in the brain. The name has been expanded to include hyperactivity, hence the H in ADHD. Now, there is also ADHD with residuals, meaning bipolar symptoms.

The ADD drug market is valued at four billion dollars annually and is one of the most rapidly growing drug markets there is.[4, 5]

ADD is the number-one reason children are referred to doctors for a psychological reason.[6] According to the Centers for Disease Control and Prevention (CDC) ten percent of children have been diagnosed with this disorder.[7] Some of the symptoms include difficulty concentrating, inability to sit still, behavioral problems, irritability, hyperactivity, impulsiveness and mood swings.

Many symptoms of ADD are identical to those of nutritional imbalance. In fact, data has shown diet interventions have a better than 70 percent success rate in treating ADD[8], but very few ever receive nutritional treatment; instead, millions of children are being prescribed powerful stimulants and other medications.[9]

Studies have implicated food additives, refined sugars, food sensitivities or allergies, and fatty acids in ADD.[10]

Amphetamines are most often prescribed for ADD. These drugs have a similar chemical structure to, and same addictive qualities of, cocaine.[11]

Despite being the most commonly prescribed medications, they are not very effective. Forty-two percent of those treated with stimulant medication do not respond as intended and some even show increased behavior problems.

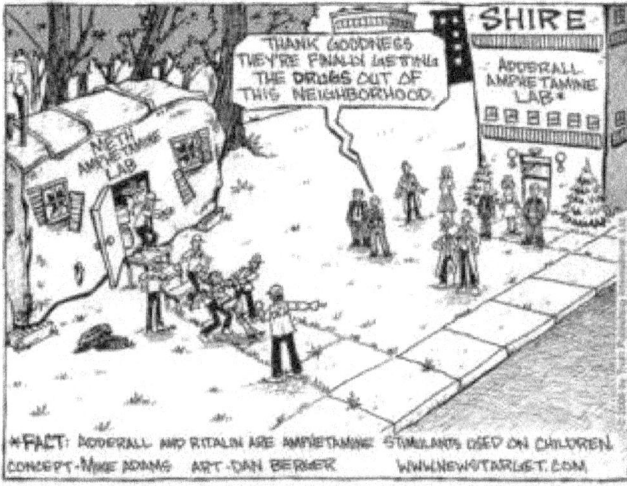

COUNTERTHINK

SHIRE

THANK GOODNESS THEY'RE FINALLY GETTING THE DRUGS OUT OF THIS NEIGHBORHOOD.

METH AMPHETAMINE LAB

ADDERALL AMPHETAMINE LAB*

*FACT: ADDERALL AND RITALIN ARE AMPHETAMINE STIMULANTS USED ON CHILDREN.
CONCEPT-MIKE ADAMS   ART-DAN BERGER   WWW.NEWSTARGET.COM

Some of the side effects of amphetamine medications include insomnia, decreased appetite, stomachache, headache, dizziness, sadness, unhappiness, crying, picking at the skin, irritability, nightmares, tics, weight loss, reduced growth, agitation, anxiousness, psychosis, Tourette's syndrome, cognitive impairment, hypertension, hyperthyroidism, cardiovascular problems, fatal liver damage and glaucoma.

Antidepressants are also commonly prescribed for ADD. Some side effects include constipation, drowsiness, increased blood pressure, blurred vision, dry mouth, hyperactivity, nausea, facial rash, feeling "spaced out", cardiac toxicity and sudden death.

Anti-hypertensives are also used to treat ADD. Side effects include sedation, irritability, headaches, stomachaches, cardiac changes, and drops in blood pressure and heart rate.[6]

Drugs prescribed for ADD are often "gateway" drugs. Many children chop up their pills and snort them and end up using illegal drugs in later years. Prescribing medications for a disorder we do not understand is not an ideal solution and sends the wrong message to our children — that drugs are the answer.

Some experts say funding should be directed towards research on alternative therapies and it may be problematic that those making decisions about drug treatment, parents, doctors and teachers, are the same ones who appear to get the greatest benefit from it.[6]

I have talked to many parents of children with ADD and none of them *want* their child to have to take drugs. They are usually thrilled to hear diet may be a contributing factor—maybe even the cause—and wonder why no one has ever suggested this to them before. Many educators believe poor diets contribute to students' learning and behavior problems, but teachers can't do much about it.

It is time to acknowledge the benefits of nutrition in mental illness as these treatments are milder, less expensive, often more effective and lead to many more positive "side" effects than drugs. Dangerous medications should be used as a *last* and not a *first* resort.

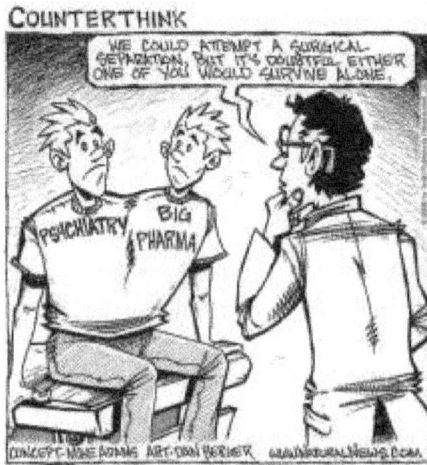

Chapter Eleven

The Cafeteria

"The destiny of nations depends on how they nourish themselves." — Jean Anthelme Brillat-Savarin

Abraham Maslow's famous model of Hierarchy of Needs states that, unless an individual's needs are met, they cannot progress to achieve higher goals of self-actualization. One who is self-actualized is able to concentrate on resolving social issues, like hunger or poverty, instead of focusing only on his or her own immediate needs.

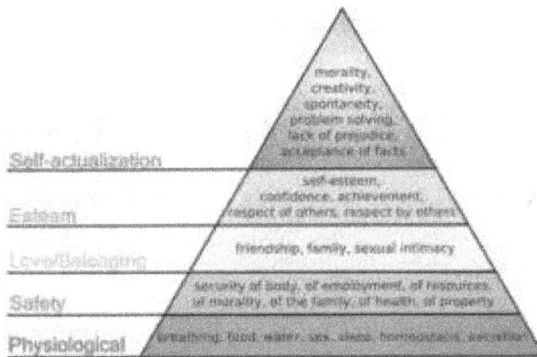

Abraham Maslow's Hierarchy of Needs

Maslow saw human beings' needs arranged like a ladder, with the most basic needs at the bottom. Maslow felt that, if the needs at the lower rungs of the ladder were unfulfilled, the person would not be able to climb to the next steps. Peak experiences occur when a person has reached the top of the ladder. These include profound moments of understanding, happiness and love, including feeling more alive, self-sufficient, whole, part of the world and more aware of truth, justice, harmony and goodness.[1]

According to Maslow's theory, lack of sufficient water or food will prevent a person from progressing toward higher levels of achievement.

In nutrition, "food security" means access by all people at all times to sufficient culturally acceptable, nutritionally adequate food through non-emergency sources.[2]

The National School Lunch Program feeds roughly 31 million children every day.[3] Many of these children come from poor areas and from families with low incomes. School meals are a great opportunity to reach children, especially those nutritionally at risk.

Studies show children who eat school meals have better behavior, attendance and academic performance. These study results were even better when the students ate both breakfast and lunch.[4] Still, many schools do not have a breakfast program and some administrators want to cut the lunch program altogether.

Meal Quality

The U.S. Centers for Disease Control states that 17 percent of children ages six to nineteen are now overweight. However, only one in four elementary schools and one in twelve high schools met the requirements for fat content in their school lunches.[5] It is important that our children eat, but also that they eat a quality meal with all of the nutrients needed to function and learn.

Unfortunately, most schools in the U.S. are similar to the one focused on in the movie *Supersize Me*. Like many school cafeterias, this North Virginia cafeteria serves a lot of processed food that is high in sugar, fat and salt and low in nutritional value.[6]

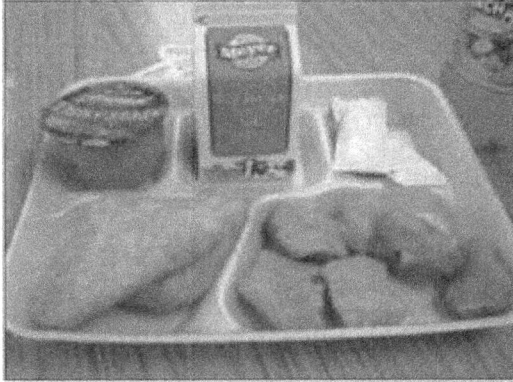

Standard U.S. School Fare

Some school cafeterias are trying to move toward healthier options, and some food-service departments are having a hard time meeting their budgets. Schools are strapped for cash, and funding is continually being cut. U.S. schools were reimbursed $2.57 for each free meal served in the 2008-09 school year and the cost was actually $2.91.

"In the past 15 years we have been changing what we sell—reducing portion sizes, meeting calorie levels, reducing fats and saturated fats," says Katie Wilson, president of the School Nutrition Association. "It's the perfect storm. We are all being required to meet nutrient standards, but the federal government is not giving us the revenue to support it."

Some districts, including the Los Angeles Unified School District in California, are trying to use their buying power to bargain for lower prices.

To save money, some schools prepare things in bulk themselves—like breakfast bars and breads. In Oregon's Portland Public Schools, they buy locally produced items like pizza with lower fat cheese and whole-grain products.[5]

In Berkeley, CA, cafeterias offer fresh, locally grown, low-fat, and low-sugar alternatives to unhealthy foods many cafeterias now serve. This idealistic program costs $4.50 per meal.

At one Berkeley middle school, they don't serve the regular school fare such as frozen pizza, fries or anything with preservatives. Instead, they serve freshly prepared, locally grown and organic food. They serve lots of fruits and vegetables and healthy versions of pizza and macaroni and cheese using ingredients like low-fat cheeses and local organic milk. The kids love the food and learn healthy food can taste good.

According to the executive chef for Berkeley Unified, in order to have a healthy meals program, it "takes a community that demands real food that is healthy, nutritious and sustainable in their communities and they have to stand up for it and they have to stand up and make a lot of noise about it."[7]

The results in Berkeley, and other schools like it, are healthier kids who don't get sick as often, have better behavior and perform better in class.[6]

There are some food experts who believe spending as little as $1 more per meal could shift cafeteria food to freshly prepared nutrient-rich foods.[8]

Some studies show improving the nutritional value of school food doesn't cost anything. A fourteen-year study showed that even though the nutritional requirements for school food went up during this time, costs did not.[9]

The common denominator in all of these programs is having *the will* to provide healthy food to students. From no added cost to one or two dollars more, we *can* serve healthier food in schools and improve children's health and education. By providing healthy food in cafeterias, administrators will be setting the right example as to what the children should be eating and students will be more likely to achieve higher goals like success and self-actualization.

Chapter Twelve

Education

"Knowledge is power." – Sir Francis Bacon

Obesity rates have doubled in children over the past 20 years. Incidences of adolescent type II diabetes have increased ten-fold in ten years.[1, 2] These and other health epidemics can be attributed to a lack of proper nutrition education.[3]

Studies show nutrition education leads to better health, yet we don't have a comprehensive nutrition education program in the U.S. Food is the base of our body chemistry and determines our body function, yet most people are performing these important experiments as untrained chemists.

We need to improve nutrition education programs in the U.S., but we cannot just add to public school curriculum without looking at the overall system, which is struggling, and often even failing, right now.[4]

Public education is overloaded with politics, inefficiency and frustrated educators. Teachers are continually being asked to take on more duties and "teach to the test". "Teaching used to be a creative and fun way to make a living," says a 35-year elementary school teacher, "but now, there is so much pressure on and demonization of teachers, that the joy of learning has been lost in the pursuit of test scores."

The textbook industry is a multi-billion-dollar industry and is, no doubt, contributing to the cost inefficiency in education. Teachers have to "follow the script" and use only assigned textbooks, which are constantly being updated and new copies purchased with every change.

There are over fifteen-thousand school districts in the U.S. This is fifteen-thousand attempts at recreating the wheel, so to speak. There are layers of state and federal departments that add to the bureaucracy.

Meanwhile, teachers are being laid off, class sizes are continually increasing and schools are in disrepair or are closing.

The amount of bureaucracy in public education may be due to a lack of running "lean", as many companies in the private sector have to do in order to survive in a competitive marketplace. Privatizing education isn't the answer, but making the system more efficient and effective is. Private corporations often must be shrewd, and since education is a basic human right, privatizing public education will likely not solve all of our problems—only change them to different ones.

Most agree there is a problem—and whatever the solution, it must be focused on to be fixed. Working, efficient models for educating our kids surely exist and they should be found and implemented.

Many children today either aren't learning or drop out of school altogether. This leads to lower education levels and limited job opportunities.

Many children without an education end up in the correctional system. One in 31 people are now in the U.S. correctional system. The U.S. has five percent of the world's population but 25 percent of its inmates.[5]

An individual without a proper education is more likely to end up on welfare. The U.S. spends roughly the same amount on welfare as it spends on education.[6, 7] We *have* to adjust our priorities.

Education is not a luxury we cannot afford and if we remain on our current path, our society will only get sicker, become less educated and productive, and the costs to society will continue to increase.

Preventative measures like education can help reverse the cycles of failure we are currently in. A change in philosophy—away from reaction and failure toward prevention and success—will save a lot of money, including on healthcare, prison, welfare and war. Everyone on this planet should receive a proper education and this includes a nutrition education. But first, we must collectively decide that failure is no longer an option.

Nutrition Education

I hear people say, "Everyone knows how to eat; they just don't want to." Nutritionists advise patients how to eat healthy for all of the reasons they learned in school. Since not everyone learns about nutrition, however, not everyone "knows how to eat." That is abundantly clear when you look at the health of our society's members.

Most adults in this country are not proficient in matters affecting their health. There are 75 million people in this country who have basic or below basic health literacy — the degree to which an individual has the capacity to process, obtain and understand basic health information and services needed to make appropriate decisions regarding their health. It is estimated that 50 to 70 billion dollars of our healthcare costs can be attributed to a low level of health literacy.[3]

The majority of public school nutrition education focuses primarily on the USDA food guide pyramid. Less than half of schools thoroughly cover topics such as the relationship between diet and health, which is what research shows really works.[8] And even though the topic predominantly covered in the classrooms that offer nutrition education is the food pyramid, only two percent of U.S. children ages two to nineteen eat a diet consistent with it.[9]

Research reveals that the instructional materials and techniques being used to teach nutrition are ineffective. Studies also show the amount of time devoted to the topic is not sufficient to create dietary changes.[10] Schools that have a coordinated nutrition program provide a more focused message about the importance of healthy eating and have better success. However, most U.S. schools have no such program.[8]

There *are* successful nutrition education programs, however. The Edible Schoolyard in Berkeley, CA, for instance, incorporates classroom instruction, gardening and cooking into the studies of math, science, history and reading.[11]

Garden nutrition education programs are a great way to teach students about nutrition and, as I mentioned in earlier chapters, they work.

School gardening increases the willingness of children to eat a wider range of fruits and vegetables. Students who participate in garden nutrition programs eat three times more fruits and vegetables than those who do not. When kids grow it, they want to eat it.[12, 13]

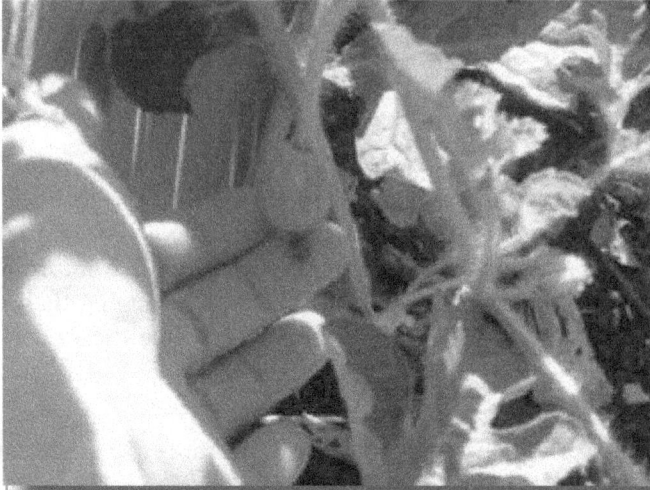

Watermelon in My School Garden

School gardens are also good for children's mental health. Researchers found just five minutes each day of an activity like gardening can boost mood and self-esteem. School gardens also improve children's development, teach life skills and make them healthier and happier.[14]

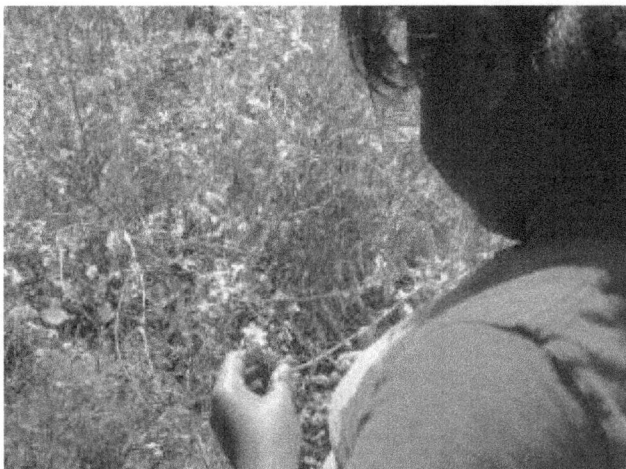
My Student Explores the Garden

It is ideal to incorporate nutrition education into preschool through 12th-grade programs, but there are other methods to gain a nutrition education when there is no such program available. Ultimately, there should be a comprehensive nutrition education program in *every* K-12 public school in the U.S.; however, this will take time. In the meantime, adults and children without access to an adequate nutrition education program can, and should be able to—through health insurance and other means (including publicly supported ones)—get this information elsewhere, like through individual nutrition consulting or free nutrition classes.

The answer to many of our health and other problems is for all people to know how to feed their bodies. The key to accomplishing this is through increased awareness, which will lead to more demand for and access to affordable, healthy food, nutrition professionals and nutrition education. This reparative formula will lead to a healthier, more productive populace, better able to reach self-actualization and contribute to the greater good of the world. These solutions address root causes of problems and solve them through education—the ultimate solution to just about *any* problem.

Developing a problem-solving approach like this was not that difficult, and we already know solutions like education and proper nutrition work, so why haven't we fixed our massive problems yet? Because an effective strategy—one that deals with the insidious resistance put up by an often invisible, self-serving, frequently wealthy, opposition that is interested in maintaining perpetual cycles of failure and the status quo—has not been developed or implemented on a wide scale. That resistance depends on the public's apathy, so spread the word and help raise awareness. If we start addressing these problems at their origins, which, as Maslow pointed out are often security related, we can remedy the world's problems. And why not?

The Power of Education

Unless someone knows why they should do something, they are likely not interested and, therefore, probably won't do it. I had one client, who we will call Leo. Leo was eleven years old and overweight. His favorite foods were sodas, chicken strips, baked potatoes with sour cream and other fatty foods. Leo never ate breakfast. I told him he must start to eat breakfast, but he stared blankly into space. I explained, without breakfast, his body and metabolism would remain in the "off" position. I also told him his body was storing fat like a chipmunk stores food in their cheeks for the long periods without food. He then appeared interested and, the next morning, Leo ate breakfast. His mother was shocked and thrilled. I was happy, too, that education had yet again proven to be an effective tool and changed this boy's life.

At the elementary school where I teach nutrition, I am often sent students who refuse to eat and who have eating disorders. Upon each student's arrival to my office, I offer them food. So far, everybody has refused it initially. But, after we discuss why they won't eat and I explain what nutrients do, each student has proceeded to eat the food I offered. All have left my office with handfuls of produce. Education works.

Doing something because you are told to is difficult. Doing something because you understand why you should is easy. Success comes when you *want* to do something, not because you feel you *have* to. If you understand nutrition, you will be motivated and will want to eat healthier; therefore, you will be successful.

This is the power of a nutrition education; and it also changed *my* life.

The difference between receiving an education and being told what to do is best described by the famous saying, "Give a man a fish and he eats for a day. Teach him to fish and he eats for a lifetime." Right now there are people who want to hand us polluted, rotting fish out of a dirty sea. We must learn to fish in a fresh new ocean.

So go on, warrior! Educate the masses so we can all heal, maintain good health, prosper and save the world. Let's begin a nutrition revolution. Good luck—go forth and conquer!

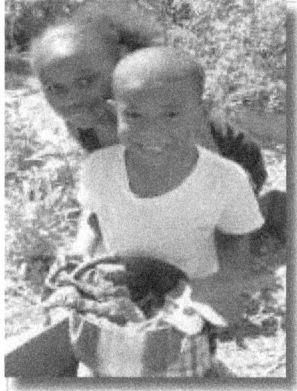

Volunteering at Oakland-Based Urban Gardens

Resources

Chapter 1, My Story

1. 48 Hours. (2001, November). Out of control. [Television series].
    San Francisco, California: CBS.

Chapter 2, Medicine

1. Warfarin. (n.d.). MedicineNet. Retrieved July 20, 2010, from
    http://www.medicinenet.com/warfarin-oral/page2.htm.
2. Kerr, G., Bloomfield, Y. (n.d.). Modern ailments ancient
    remedies: A healing manual. Smithmark.
3. Fortune Global 500 2008 — Top industries: most profitable. (2008,
    July 21). CNNMoney.com. Retrieved November 27, 2010, from
    http://money.cnn.com/magazines/fortune/global500/2008/
    performers/industries/profits/.
4. Hepp, C. (2010, November 12). Big pharma gearing up to face
    the patent cliff. The Enquirer. Retrieved January 31, 2011, from
    http://   articles.philly.com/2010-11-
    12/news/24955084_1_patentholders-patent-protection-patent-losses.
5. Smith, M. (Reporter). (n.d.). Drug companies: Too much
    influence? [Video]. (Available from Health WorldNet, Inc.,
    California). Retrieved December 12, 2009, from http://
    healthworldnet.com/Video/?C=5169.
6. Dahms, J. (2007, July). The top 10 bestselling prescription
    medicines worldwide, 200 — world's best-selling medicines. MedAd
    News.   Retrieved   November   24,   2010,   from
    http://en.wikipedia.org/wiki/List_of_bestselling_drugs.   Source
    listed as: (2007, July).
7. MedAdNews 200 — World's Best-Selling Medicines, MedAd
    News (subscription required).
8. United States Department of Agriculture. (n.d.). Background
    information and statistics: Fresh spinach. Retrieved July 20, 2010,
    from http://www.ers.usda.gov/News/spinachcoverage.htm.
9. Antithrombotics — pharma in R&D battle as warfarin goes on:
    Datamonitor study. (2005, November 21). Goliath. Retrieved January

31, 2011, from http://goliath.ecnext.com/coms2/ gi_0199-4954007/Antithrombotics-pharma-in-R-D.html.

10. United States Department of Agriculture, Economics, Statistics and Market Information System. (2010, October). Fruit and tree nut yearbook spreadsheet files. Table E-7 almonds: acreage, yield per acre, production (shelled basis), season-average grower price, and value, California to date. Retrieved November 7, 2010, from http://usda.mannlib.cornell.edu/MannUsda/ viewDocumentInfo.do?documentID=1377.

11. Erectile dysfunction: Alternative treatments. (n.d.). Web MD. Retrieved July 20, 2010, from http://www.webmd.com/ erectile-dysfunction/guide/alternative-treatments-ed.

12. Wong, C. (2007, September 21). Natural remedies for erectile dysfunction. About, Alternative Medicine. Retrieved July 20, 2010, from http://altmedicine.about.com/cs/conditionsetoh/a/ erectiledysfunc.htm.

13. Kennedy, V.B. (2009, October 20). Pfizer, Inc. reported a 26% spike in third-quarter profit early Tuesday, helped by lower expenses and charges taken in the 2008 quarter for litigation. Marketwatch. Retrieved November 27, 2009, from http://www. marketwatch.com/story/pfizer-reports-26-higher-profit-butlower-sales-2009-10-20.

14. Lakhan, S.E., Vieira, K.F. (2008). Nutritional therapies for mental disorders. Nutrition Journal, 7:2 doi: 10.1186/1475-2891-7-2, online at: http://www.nutritionj.com/content/7/1/2.

15. Wilson, K.B. (2010, April). California Healthcare Almanac: health care costs 101. California Healthcare Foundation. Retrieved November 19, 2010, from http://www.chcf.org/~/media/Files/ PDF/H/PDF%20HealthCareCosts10.pdf.

16. Henry J. Kaiser Foundation. (2009, March 18). Health care costs: A primer. Retrieved January 31, 2011, from http://www.kff.org/ insurance/upload/7670_02.pdf.

17. Mateljan, G. (2009, June 24). Open letter to President Barack Obama. World's Healthiest Foods. Retrieved December 12, 2009, from http://whfoods.org/genpage.php?tname=george&dbid=249.

18. How to get insurance coverage for dietary counseling. (2005). MedicineNet. Retrieved December 1, 2009, from http://www. medicinenet.com/script/main/art.asp?articlekey=50695&pf=3& page=1.

19. Neel, J. (2009, June 9). Medical schools and drug firm dollars. NPR: Health and Science. Retrieved October 1, 2009, from

http://www. npr.org/templates/story/story.php?storyId=4696316&sc=emaf.

20. Adams, K.M., Lindell, K.C., Kohlmeier, M., Zeisel, S.H. (2006, April). Status of nutrition education in medical schools. American Journal of Clinical Nutrition, 83(4):941S–944S.

21. Kamen, B. (Actor), Grapek, J.H. (Director). (2004). ADD/ADHD smart solutions: Ways to improve your child's behavior. [Video]. (Available from Associated Producers, Inc., Bethesda, Maryland).

22. Olbermann, K. (Interviewer). (2010, November 17). Interview of Wendell Potter former CIGNA executive and author of "Deadly Spin". [Television broadcast interview]. New York: MSNBC.

23. Sahelian, R. (n.d.). Quackwatch review. Retrieved July 20, 2010, from http://www.raysahelian.com/quackwatch.html.

24. Eisen, S.C. (2005, October 13). Quackwatch founder Stephen Barrett loses major defamation trial in hometown. Foundation for Health Choice. Retrieved December 15, 2009, from http://www. foundationforhealthchoice.com/victory_barett.html.

25. Dilanian, K. (2007, May 11). Senators who weakened drug bill got millions from industry. USA Today. Retrieved December 12, 2009, from http://www.usatoday.com/news/washington/200705-10-senators-drug-bill_N.htm.

26. Donohue, J., Cevasco, M., Rosenthal, M. (2007, August). A decade of direct-to-consumer advertising of prescription drugs. New England Journal of Medicine, 357:673-681.

27. Moynihan, R., Henry, D. (2006, April). The fight against disease mongering: Generating knowledge for action. Public Library of Science Medicine, 3(4).

28. Walker, M. (2003). German cancer therapies (pg. 108). New York: Kensington Publishing Group.

Chapter 3, Society

1. Campbell, C. (2001, August 21). Health education behaviors models and theories—a review of the literature part 1. Mississippi State University, Coordinated Access to the Research and Extension System (C.A.R.E.S.). Retrieved October 2009, from http://msucares.com/health/health/appa1.htm.

2. Chilton, M., Chyatte, M., Breaux, J. (2007, October). The effects of poverty and food insecurity on child development. Indian J Med Res, 126:262-272.

3.   Food fight: childhood obesity and the food industry. (2003, July 17). Nightline. [Television series]. New York, New York: ABC.

4.   Baertlein, L. (2010, November 12). San Francisco mayor to veto curb on fast-food toys. Reuters. Retrieved February 3, 2011, from http://www.reuters.com/article/2010/11/12/us-fastfood-toysidUSTRE6AB4UG20101112?sp=true.

5.   Reisner, R. (n.d.). The diet industry: A big fat lie. Business Week. Retrieved December 28, 2009, from http://www.businessweek. com/debateroom/archives/2008/03/the_diet_indust.html.

6.   Reece, E.A. (2009, February 8). Legislators: Stimulate the economy with biomedical research. The Baltimore Examiner. Retrieved November 24, 2010, from http://www.umbi.umd.edu/ news/2009/images/090209_examiner.pdf.

7.   Wilson, K.B. (2010, April). California Healthcare Almanac: health care costs 101. California Healthcare Foundation. Retrieved November 19, 2010, from http://www.chcf.org/~/media/Files/ PDF/H/PDF%20HealthCareCosts10.pdf.

8.   Webb hearing explores cost of incarceration in the United States. (2007, October 4). Retrieved July 20, 2010, from http://webb. senate.gov/newsroom/pressreleases/2007-10-04-03.cfm.

9.   Chantrill, C. Welfare Spending. U.S. Government Spending. Retrieved January 6, 2011, from http://www. usgovernmentspending.com/welfare_chart_40.html.

10. Wolf. R. (2010, May 13). Afghan war costs now outpace Iraq's 100 billion a year from 2002 through 2010. USA Today. Retrieved November 20, 2010, from http://www.usatoday.com/ news/military/2010-05-12-afghan_N.htm.

11. U.S. Department of Education, National Center for Education Statistics. (2009). Revenues and expenditures for public elementary and secondary education: School year 2006–07 (fiscal year 2007). Retrieved March 16, 2009, from http://nces.ed.gov/ pubs2009/2009337.pdf.

12. Jewsbury, M., Owen, J. (2010, June 27). School gardeners perform better in the classroom. The Independent. Retrieved October 9, 2010, from http://www.independent.co.uk/life-style/ house-and-home/gardening/school-gardeners-perform-better-inthe-classroom-2011528.html.

13. United States Department of Agriculture, Agriculture Research Service. Phytoremediation: Using plants to clean up soils. Retrieved December 16, 2010, from http://www.ars.usda.gov/is/ AR/archive/jun00/soil0600.htm.

14. Raskin, I. (n.d.). Phytoremediation: Using plants to remove pollutants from the environment. American Society of Plant Biologists. Retrieved February 1, 2011, from http://www.aspb.org/publicaffairs/briefing/phytoremediation.cfm.

Chapter 4, Politics

1.   Interview of former Goldman Sachs bank executive and author of "It Takes a Pillage" Naomi Prins. (2009, December 21). [Television broadcast interview]. Atlanta, Georgia: CNN.
2.   Comstock, C. (2010, June 30). Former SEC whistleblower Gary Aguirre gets vindication for his pursuit of John Mack.
3.   Business Insider. Retrieved December 2, 2010, from http://www. businessinsider.com/aguirre-sec-john-mack-pequot-2010-6.
4.   Adams, M. (2009, January 12). FDA is deeply "corrupted and distorted," claim its own scientists in protest letter. Natural News. Retrieved January 13, 2009, from http://www.naturalnews.com/News_000655_FDA_scientists_Obama_corruption.html.
5.   Ismael, M.A. (2005, July 7). FDA: A shell of its former self "The food and drug administration lacks the power to regulate pharmaceuticals and keep you safe." The Center for Public Integrity. Retrieved December 12, 2009, from http://projects.publicintegrity.org/rx//report.aspx?aid=722.
6.   Donohue, J., Cevasco, M., Rosenthal, M. (2007, August). A decade of direct-to-consumer advertising of prescription drugs. New England Journal of Medicine, 357:673-681.
7.   Center for Responsive Politics. (2010, April 25). Lobbying spending database. Retrieved July 20, 2010, from http://www.opensecrets.org/lobby/top.php?showYear=a&indexType=i.
8.   Moore, M. (Director). (2007). Sicko. [Video]. Dog Eat Dog Films, Inc.

Chapter 5, Amino Acids

1.   Mindell, E. (1999). Vitamin bible for the 21st century. New York: Warner Books.
2.   Balch, P.A. (2006). Prescription for nutritional healing (4th ed.). New York: Avery Publishing.

3. Erectile dysfunction: Alternative treatments. (n.d.). Web MD. Retrieved July 20, 2010, from http://www.webmd.com/ erectile-dysfunction/guide/alternative-treatments-ed.

4. Wong, C. (2007, September 21). Natural remedies for erectile dysfunction. About, Alternative Medicine. Retrieved July 20, 2010, from http://altmedicine.about.com/cs/conditionsetoh/a/ erectiledysfunc.htm.

5. Lakhan, S.E., Vieira, K.F. (2008). Nutritional therapies for mental disorders. Nutrition Journal, 7:2 doi: 10.1186/1475-2891-7-2, online at: http://www.nutritionj.com/content/7/1/2.

6. Taurine. (n.d.). eMedTV. Retrieved July 20, 2010, from http:// congestive-heart-failure.emedtv.com/taurine/taurine.html.

7. Mahan, L.K., Escott-Stump, S. (2004). Krause's food, nutrition & diet therapy (11th ed.). St. Louis, Missouri: Saunders/Elsevier.

8. Grosvenor, M., Smolin, L. (2002). Nutrition, from science to life. Florida: Harcourt, Inc.

9. Self Nutrition Data. (n.d.). Know what you eat. Retrieved April 4, 2011, from http://nutritiondata.self.com.

Chapter 6, Micronutrients

1. National Institutes of Health. (n.d.). Vitamins: Medlineplus. Retrieved July 20, 2010, from www.nlm.nih.gov/medlineplus/ vitamins.html.

2. Grosvenor, M., Smolin, L. (2002). Nutrition, from science to life. Florida: Harcourt, Inc.

3. Balch, J.F., Balch P.A. (1997). Prescription for nutritional healing (2nd ed.). New York: Avery Publishing Group.

4. Balch, P.A. (2006). Prescription for nutritional healing (4th ed.). New York: Avery Publishing.

5. Self Nutrition Data. (n.d.). Know what you eat. Retrieved December 27, 2009, from http://www.nutritiondata.com/ foods-0.html.

6. United States Department of Health and Human Services and United States Department of Agriculture. (2010). Dietary guidelines for Americans. Retrieved February 3, 2011, from http:// www.cnpp.usda.gov/Publications/DietaryGuidelines/2010/ PolicyDoc/PolicyDoc.pdf.

Chapter 7, Macronutrients

1.   Balch, P.A. (2006). Prescription for nutritional healing (4th ed.). New York: Avery Publishing.
2.   Balch, J.F., Balch P.A. (1997). Prescription for nutritional healing (2nd ed.). New York: Avery Publishing Group.
3.   Grosvenor, M., Smolin, L. (2002). Nutrition, from science to life. Florida: Harcourt, Inc.
4.   Self Nutrition Data. (n.d.). Know what you eat. Retrieved December 27, 2009, from http://www.nutritiondata.com/ foods-0.html.
5.   United States Department of Health and Human Services and United States Department of Agriculture. (2010). Dietary guidelines for Americans. Retrieved February 3, 2011 from http://www.cnpp.usda.gov/Publications/DietaryGuidelines/2010/PolicyDoc/PolicyDoc.pdf.
6.   State of the air. (2010). American Lung Association. Retrieved November 20, 2010, from http://www.stateoftheair.org/2010/ key-findings.

Chapter 8, Diet

1. United States Department of Agriculture. (2009). National nutrient database for standard reference, release 22. Retrieved December 30, 2009, from http://www.nal.United States Department of Agriculture.gov/fnic/foodcomp/search/.

Chapter 9, Research

1.   Grosvenor, M., Smolin, L. (2002). Nutrition, from science to life. Florida: Harcourt, Inc.
2.   Neel, J. (2009, June 9). Medical schools and drug firm dollars. NPR: Health and Science. Retrieved October 1, 2009, from http://www. npr.org/templates/story/story.php?storyId=4696316&sc=emaf.
3.   Perlis, R.H., Perlis, C.S., Wu, Y., Hwang, C., Joseph, M., Nierenberg, A.A. (2005, October). Industry sponsorship and financial conflict of interest in the reporting of clinical trials in psychiatry. American Journal of Psychiatry, 162(10):1957-60.

4. Bateman, B., Warner, J.O., Hutchinson, E., Dean, T., Rowlandson, P., Gant, C., Grundy, J., Fitzgerald, C., Stevenson, J. (2004, June). The effects of a double-blind, placebo controlled, artificial food colourings and benzoate preservative challenge on hyperactivity in a general population sample of preschool children. Arch Dis Child, 89(6):506-11.

5. Carter, C.M., Urbanowicz, M., Hemsley, R., Mantilla, L., Strobel, S., Graham, P.J., Taylor, E. (1993, November). Effects of a few food diet in attention deficit disorder. Arch Dis Child, 69(5):564-8.

6. Doggett, M.A. (2004). ADHD and drug therapy: Is it still a valid treatment? Journal of Child Health Care, 8(1):69-81.

7. Boris, M., Mandel, F.S. (1994, May). Foods and additives are common causes of the attention deficit hyperactive disorder in children. Ann Allergy, 72(5):462-8.

8. Akhondzadeh, S., Mohammadi, M., Khademi, M. (2004, April 8). Zinc sulfate as an adjunct to methylphenidate for the treatment of attention deficit hyperactivity disorder in children. B.M.C. Psychiatry, 4:9.

9. Otero, G., Pliego-Rivero, F.B., Contreras, J.R., Fernandez, T. (2004, July 25). Iron supplementation brings up a lacking P300 in iron deficient children. Clinical Neuropsychology, 115(10):2259-2266.

10. Young, S.N. (2002, January 22). Clinical nutrition 3: The fuzzy boundary between nutrition and psychopharmacology. CMAJ, 166(2):205–209. Retrieved November 25, 2010, from http://www.ncbi.nlm.nih.gov/pmc/articles/PMC99276/?tool=pubmed.

11. Meyers, S. (2000). Use of neurotransmitter precursors for treatment of depression. Alternative Medicine Review, 5(1):64-71.

12. Balch, P.A. (2006). Prescription for nutritional healing (4th ed.). New York: Avery Publishing.

13. Llewellyn, D.J., Langa, K.M., Lang, I.A. (2009, September). Serum 25-hydroxyvitamin D concentration and cognitive impairment. U.K. Journal of Geriatric Psychiatry, Neurology, 22(3):188-95.

14. Tveden-Nyborg, P., Johansen, L.K., Raida, Z., et al. (2009, September). Vitamin C deficiency in early postnatal life impairs spatial memory and reduces the number of hippocampal neurons in guinea pigs. American Journal of Clinical Nutrition, 90(3):540-6.

15. Lakhan, S.E., Vieira, K.F. (2008). Nutritional therapies for mental disorders. Nutrition Journal, 7:2 doi: 10.1186/1475-2891-7-2, online at: http://www.nutritionj.com/content/7/1/2.

16. Potential weight-loss effects of African mango. (2009, April). The Natural Standard Research Collaboration. Retrieved December 12, 2009, from http://naturalstandard.com.

17. Folic acid may improve asthma, allergies. (2009, May). The Natural Standard Research Collaboration. Retrieved December 12, 2009, from http://naturalstandard.com.

18. Tabak, C., Wijga, A.H., de Meer, G., Janssen, N.A.H., Brunekreef, B., Smit, H.A. (2005, October 21). Diet and asthma in Dutch school children. Thorax, 20`06, 61(12):1048–1053. Published online, doi: 10.1136/thx.2005.043034. Retrieved December 12, 2009, from http://www.ncbi.nlm.nih.gov/pmc/articles/PMC2117046/?report=abstract.

19. Vitamin C may affect blood pressure. (2009, January). The Natural Standard Research Collaboration. Retrieved December 12, 2009, from http://naturalstandard.com.

20. Algae for blood clots. (2007, August). The Natural Standard Research Collaboration. Retrieved December 12, 2009, from http://naturalstandard.com.

21. Acupuncture for blood pressure. (2007, August). The Natural Standard Research Collaboration. Retrieved December 12, 2009, from http://naturalstandard.com/news/news200708006.asp.

22. Phytoestrogens for bone health. (2007, August). The Natural Standard Research Collaboration. Retrieved December 12, 2009, from http://naturalstandard.com.

23. Morley, K.L., Ferguson, P.J., Koropatnick, J. (2007, June 18). Tangeretin and nobiletin induce G1 cell cycle arrest but not apoptosis in human breast and colon cancer cells. Cancer Lett, 251(1):168-78.

24. Foltz-Gray, D. (2003, Jan., Feb.). Good Food—The Magic of Mushrooms. Alternative Medicine, pp. 39-45.

25. Chi-Fung Chan, G., Man-Yuen Sze, D. (2009). Supplements for immune enhancement in hematologic malignancies. Hematology, pp. 313-319. Retrieved August 5, 2010, from http://asheducationbook.hematologylibrary.org/cgi/content/full/2009/1/313.

26. Pomegranate for prostate cancer. (2009, May). The Natural Standard Research Collaboration. Retrieved December 12, 2009, from http://naturalstandard.com.

27. Shanafelt, T.D., Call, T.G., Zent, C.S., et al. (2009, May 26). Phase I trial of daily oral polyphenon E. in patients with asymptomatic rai

stage 0 to II chronic lymphocytic leukemia. Journal of Clinical Oncology, 10;27(23):3808-14.

28. Severson, K. (2010, September 24). Told to eat its vegetables, America orders fries. NY Times. Retrieved September 27, 2010, from http://www.nytimes.com/2010/09/25/health/ policy/25vegetables.html?pagewanted=1&_r=2.

29. University of California at Davis, Nutrition Department. (2006, February). Clinical nutrition course 116b: Nutrition and cancer.

30. United States Department of Agriculture, Food and Nutrition Information Center, National Agriculture Library. (2004, March). Nutrition, learning and behavior in children: A resource for professionals. Baltimore, Maryland. Retrieved April 13, 2006, from http://www.nal.UnitedStatesDepartmentofAgriculture.gov/ fnic/service/learnpub.html.

31. Foster, B.L. (2009, August 31). School-lunch staff bring nutrition to the table. Edutopia, Retrieved October 13, 2009, from www. edutopia.org/school-lunch-cafeteria-budget-nutrition.

32. United States Department of Agriculture, Expanded Food and Nutrition Education Program. (2006). Impact data. Retrieved January 13, 2009, from http://www.nifa.usda.gov/nea/food/ efnep/pdf/2006_impact.pdf.

33. Adams, K.M., Lindell, K.C., Kohlmeier, M., Zeisel, S.H. (2006, April). Status of nutrition education in medical schools. American Journal of Clinical Nutrition, 83(4):941S–944S.

34. How to get insurance coverage for dietary counseling. (2005). MedicineNet. Retrieved December 1, 2009, from http://www. medicinenet.com/script/main/art.asp?articlekey=50695&pf=3& page=1.

Chapter 10, The Brain

1. Lakhan, S.E., Vieira, K.F. (2008). Nutritional therapies for mental disorders. Nutrition Journal, 7:2 doi: 10.1186/1475-2891-7-2, online at: http://www.nutritionj.com/content/7/1/2.

2. Meyers, S. (2000). Use of neurotransmitter precursors for treatment of depression. Alternative Medicine Review, 5(1):64-71.

3. Balch, P.A. (2006). Prescription for nutritional healing (4th ed.). New York: Avery Publishing.

4.   Commercial and pipeline insight: ADHD. (n.d.). Retrieved November 28, 2010, from https://www.leaddiscovery.co.uk/reports/1055/Commercial_and_Pipeline_Insight_ADHD.

5.   ADD and ADHD drug revenues. (n.d.). Retrieved January 13, 2009, from www.leaddiscovery.co.uk.com.

6.   Doggett, M.A. (2004). ADHD and drug therapy: Is it still a valid treatment? Journal of Child Health Care, 8(1):69-81.

7.   Centers for Disease Control and Prevention. (2010, May 25). Attention deficit hyperactivity disorder: Data and statistics in the United States. Retrieved November 27, 2010, from http://www.cdc.gov/ncbddd/adhd/data.html.

8.   Lawlis, F. (2004). The ADD answer. New York: Penguin Group.

9.   Kamen, B. (Actor), Grapek, J.H. (Director). (2004). ADD/ ADHD smart solutions: Ways to improve your child's behavior. [Video]. (Available from Associated Producers, Inc., Bethesda, Maryland).

10. Schnoll, R., Burshteyn, D., Cea-Aravena, J. (2004, November 2). Nutrition in the treatment of attention deficit hyperactivity disorder: A neglected but important aspect. Applied Psychophysiology and Biofeedback, 28(1):63-75. 1090-0586 (Print) 1573-3270 (Online).

11. DeGrandpre, R. (1999). Ritalin nation. New York: W.W. Norton and Company.

Chapter 11, The Cafeteria

1.   A science odyssey, people and discoveries: Abraham Maslow. (n.d.). PBS. Retrieved July 20, 2010, from http://www.pbs.org/wgbh/aso/databank/entries/bhmasl.html.

2.   Heinig, J. (2006, February). UC Davis community nutrition course 118: Food insecurity and hunger.

3.   United States Department of Agriculture: Economic Research Service. (2010, June 14). Child nutrition programs: National school lunch program. Retrieved November 27, 2010, from http://www.ers.usda.gov/Briefing/ChildNutrition/lunch.htm.

4.   United States Department of Agriculture, Food and Nutrition Information Center, National Agriculture Library. (2004, March). Nutrition, learning and behavior in children: a resource for professionals. Baltimore, Maryland. Retrieved April 13, 2006, from http://www.nal.usda.gov/fnic/service/learning.pdf.

5.   Foster, B.L. (2009, August 31). School-lunch staff bring nutrition to the table. Edutopia, Retrieved October 13, 2009, from www.Edutopia.org/school-lunch-cafeteria-budget-nutrition.
6.   Waters, A. (2009, September 21). A forum: Food for all, how to grow democracy. The Nation, pp. 12-13. Online at: http://www.thenation.com/article/healthy-constitution.
7.   Ellis, K. and Rosenfeld, L. (Producers, Writers and Directors). (2009, August 26). A healthy school lunch. [Video]. (Available from Edutopia, San Rafael, California). Retrieved July 20, 2010, from www.edutopia.org/school-lunch-nutrition-berkeley-video.
8.   Mateljan, G. (2009, June 24). Open letter to President Barack Obama. World's Healthiest Foods. Retrieved December 12, 2009, from http://whfoods.org/genpage.php?tname=george&dbid=249.
9.   United States Department of Agriculture, Food and Nutrition Service. (n.d.). Meal cost study. Retrieved July 19, 2010, from http://www.fns.usda.gov/ora/menu/Published/CNP/FILES/MealCostStudy.pdf.

Chapter 12, Education

1.   Wooten, M., Stitizel, K. (2003). Nutrition education, a position statement. The National Alliance for Nutrition and Activity. Washington, D.C.
2.   Centers for Disease Control and Prevention. (n.d.). Diabetes and women's health across the life stages: A public health perspective. Retrieved February 3, 2011, from http://www.cdc.gov/diabetes/pubs/women/index.htm.
3.   American Association for Health Education. (2008). Health literacy. Retrieved December 9, 2009, from www.aahperd.org/ aahe.
4.   U.S. Department of Education, National Center for Education Statistics. (2009). The nations report card. Retrieved February 3, 2011, from http://nces.ed.gov/nationsreportcard/pdf/main2009/2011451.pdf.
5.   Study: 7.3 million in U.S. prison system in '07. (2009, March 2). CNN. Retrieved November 26, 2010, from http://edition.cnn.com/2009/CRIME/03/02/record.prison.population/index.html?iref=allsearch.
6.   Chantrill, C. Welfare Spending. U.S. Government Spending. Retrieved January 6, 2011, from http://www.usgovernmentspending.com/welfare_chart_40.html.

7. U.S. Department of Education, National Center for Education Statistics. (2009). Revenues and expenditures for public elementary and secondary education: School year 2006–07 (fiscal year 2007). Retrieved March 16, 2009, from http://nces.ed.gov/pubs2009/2009337.pdf.

8. U.S. Department of Education, National Center for Education Statistics. (1996). Nutrition education in public elementary and secondary schools. Retrieved April 28, 2011, from http://nces.ed.gov/pubs/web/96852.asp.

9. National Alliance for Nutrition and Activity. (2005, March). Model of local school wellness policies on physical activity and nutrition. Washington, D.C.

10. U.S. Department of Education, National Center for Education Statistics. (2000). Nutrition Education in Public School Elementary School Classrooms, K-5. Retrieved April 28, 2011, from http://nces.ed.gov/pubs2000/2000040.pdf.

11. Waters, A. (2009, September 21). A forum: Food for all, how to grow democracy. The Nation, pp. 12-13. Online at: http://www.thenation.com/article/healthy-constitution.

12. Jewsbury, M., Owen, J. (2010, June 27). School gardeners perform better in the classroom. The Independent. Retrieved October 9, 2010, from http://www.independent.co.uk/life-style/house-and-home/gardening/school-gardeners-perform-better-inthe-classroom-2011528.html.

13. Ellis, K. and Rosenfeld, L. (Producers, Writers and Directors). (2009, August 26). A healthy school lunch. [Video]. (Available from Edutopia, San Rafael, California). Retrieved July 20, 2010, from www.edutopia.org/school-lunch-nutrition-berkeley-video.

14. Ernst, J. (2010, May 2). Five minutes in the green can boost mood. Reuters. Retrieved August 5, 2010, from http://www.reuters.com/article/idUSTRE6401Y620100502.

About the Author

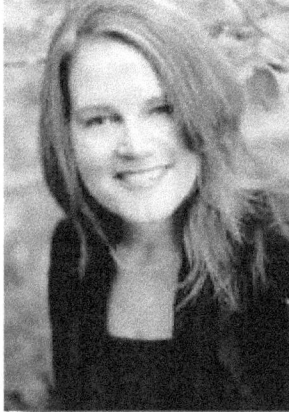

Elizabeth Kahn received her degree in clinical nutrition from the University of California at Davis. Kahn has published many health-based articles, teaches nutrition and has a private nutrition consulting practice. Kahn currently resides in the San Francisco Bay Area where she was born and raised. Connect with Elizabeth Kahn and discover other articles written by her:

A Nutrition Revolution: www.anutritionrevolution.com.

www.ingramcontent.com/pod-product-compliance
Lightning Source LLC
Chambersburg PA
CBHW030256030426
42336CB00009B/399